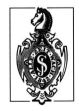

World Health Organization

The *International Histological Classification of Tumours* consists of the follow-
 [...] Each of these volumes – apart from volumes 1 and 2, which have already
[...] – will appear in a revised edition within the next few years. Volumes of
[...]ditions can be ordered through WHO, Distribution and Sales, Avenue
[...] 211 Geneva 27.

[...]cal typing of lung tumours (1967, second edition 1981)
2. [...]cal typing of breast tumours (1968, second edition 1981)
4. Histological typing of oral and oropharyngeal tumours (1971)
8. Cytology of the female genital tract (1973)
9. Histological typing of ovarian tumours (1973)
10. Histological typing of urinary bladder tumours (1973)
12. Histological typing of skin tumours (1974)
13. Histological typing of female genital tract tumours (1975)
14. Histological and cytological typing of neoplastic diseases of haematopoietic
    and lymphoid tissues (1976)
16. Histological typing of testis tumours (1977)
17. Cytology of non-gynaecological sites (1977)
20. Histological typing of tumours of the liver, biliary tract and pancreas (1978)
22. Histological typing of prostate tumours (1980)
23. Histological typing of endocrine tumours (1980)
24. Histological typing of tumours of the eye and its adnexa (1980)
25. Histological typing of kidney tumours (1981)

A coded compendium of the International Histological Classification of Tumours
(1978).

The following volumes have already appeared in a revised edition with Springer-Verlag:

Histological Typing of Thyroid Tumours, 2nd edn. Hedinger/Williams/Sobin (1988)
Histological Typing of Intestinal Tumours, 2nd edn. Jass/Sobin (1989)
Histological Typing of Oesophageal and Gastric Tumours, 2nd edn.
Watanabe/Jass/Sobin (1990)
Histological Typing of Tumours of the Gallbladder and Extrahepatic Bile Ducts,
2nd edn. Albores-Saavedra/Henson/Sobin (1990)
Histological Typing of Tumours of the Upper Respiratory Tract and Ear, 2nd edn.
Shanmugaratnam/Sobin (1991)
Histological Typing of Salivary Gland Tumours, 2nd edn. Seifert (1991)
Histological Typing of Odontogenic Tumours, 2nd edn. Kramer/Pindborg/Shear
(1992)
Histological Typing of Tumours of the Central Nervous System, 2nd edn.
Kleihues/Burger/Scheithauer (1993)
Histological Typing of Bone Tumours, 2nd edn. Schajowicz (1993)
Histological Typing of Soft Tissue Tumours, 2nd edn. Weiss (1994)

Histological Typing of Soft Tissue Tumours

S. W. Weiss

In Collaboration with L. H. Sobin
and Pathologists in 9 Countries

Second Edition

With 170 Figures

Springer-Verlag
Berlin Heidelberg New York
London Paris Tokyo
Hong Kong Barcelona
Budapest

S. W. Weiss
Professor and Director of Anatomic Pathology,
The University of Michigan Hospitals,
Ann Arbor, MI 48109-0054, USA

Series Editor
L. H. Sobin
Head, WHO Collaborating Centre
for the International Histological Classification of Tumours,
Armed Forces Institute of Pathology, Washington DC 20306, USA

First edition published by WHO in 1969 as No. 3 in the International Histological Classification of Tumours series

ISBN 3-540-56794-1 Springer-Verlag Berlin Heidelberg New York
ISBN 0-387-56794-1 Springer-Verlag New York Berlin Heidelberg

Participants

Allen, P. W., Dr.
The Queen Elizabeth Hospital, Woodville South, South Australia

Angervall, L., Dr.
Sahlgren Hospital, Göteborg, Sweden

Enjoji, M., Dr.
Kyushu University Faculty of Medicine, Fukuoka, Japan

Enzinger, F., Dr.
Bethesda, Maryland, USA

Llombart-Bosch, A., Dr.
Catedratico Medicina, Valencia, Spain

Mandard, A. M., Dr.
Centre Regional Francois Baclesse, Caen, France

Meister, P., Dr.
Institut für Pathologie, Munich, FRG

Moebius, G., Dr.
Pathologisches Institut, Bezirkskrankenhaus Schwerin, FRG

Ninfo, V., Dr.
Universita di Padova Cattedra di Anatomia e Istologia
Pathologia III, Padua, Italy

Sobin, L. H., Dr.
Armed Forces Institute of Pathology, Washington, DC, USA

Weiss, S. W., Dr.
University of Michigan Medical Center, Ann Arbor, Michigan, USA

Zhang, R-Y., Dr.
Cancer Hospital, Shanghai Medical University, Shanghai, People's
Republic of China

General Preface to the Series

Among the prerequisites for comparative studies of cancer is international agreement on histological criteria for the definition and classification of cancer types and a standardized nomenclature. An internationally agreed classification of tumours, acceptable alike to physicians, surgeons, radiologists, pathologists and statisticians, would enable cancer workers in all parts of the world to compare their findings and would facilitate collaboration among them.

In a report published in 1952,[1] a subcommittee of the World Health Organization (WHO) Expert Committee on Health Statistics discussed the general principles that should govern the statistical classification of tumours and agreed that, to ensure the necessary flexibility and ease of coding, three separate classifications were needed according to (1) anatomical site, (2) histological type, and (3) degree of malignancy. A classification according to anatomical site is available in the International Classification of Diseases.[2]

In 1956, the WHO Executive Board passed a resolution[3] requesting the Director-General to explore the possibility that WHO might organize centres in various parts of the world and arrange for the collection of human tissues and their histological classification. The main purpose of such centres would be to develop histological definitions of cancer types and to facilitate the wide adoption of a uniform nomenclature. The resolution was endorsed by the Tenth World Health Assembly in May, 1957.[4]

---

[1] WHO (1952) WHO Technical Report Series. No. 53, 1952, p 45
[2] WHO (1977) Manual of the international statistical classification of diseases, injuries, and causes of death. 1975 version Geneva
[3] WHO (1956) WHO Official Records. No. 68, p 14 (resolution EB 17.R 40)
[4] WHO (1957) WHO Official Records. No. 79, p 467 (resolution WHA 10.18)

Since 1958, WHO has established a number of centres concerned with this subject. The result of this endeavour has been the *International Histological Classification of Tumours,* a multivolumed series whose first edition was published between 1967 and 1981. The present revised second edition aims to update the classification, reflecting progress in diagnosis and the relevance of tumour types to clinical and epidemiological features.

Preface to Histological Typing
of Soft Tissue Tumours, Second Edition

The first edition of *Histological Typing of Soft Tissue Tumours*[1] was
the result of a collaborative effort organized by WHO and carried out
by the International Reference/Collaborating Centre for the Histological Classification of Soft Tissue Tumours at the Armed Forces
Institute of Pathology, Washington, D. C., United States of America.
The Centre was established in 1958 and the classification published in
1969.

In order to keep the classification current, a new group of partici-
pants was appointed in 1988 which coordinated its activities from the
University of Michigan School of Medicine, United States of America. Over the ensuing 4 years, the group met regularly at the United
States-Canadian Academy of Pathology meetings and eventually
drafted the present classification which was presented in its final
form at the International Academy of Pathology Congress in
Madrid, Spain in October 1992.

The histological classification of soft tissue tumours, which ap-
pears on pages 7–14, contains the morphology code numbers of the
International Classification of Diseases for Oncology (ICD-O)[2] and
the Systematized Nomenclature of Medicine (SNOMED).[3]

This classification, of course, reflects the present state of knowl-
edge, and modifications will certainly be needed as experience accu-
mulates and technological advances are incorporated into the daily
practice of pathology. Although the present classification represents

---

[1] Enzinger FM, Lattes R, Torloni H (1969) Histological typing of soft tissue
tumours. World Health Organization, Geneva (International Histological
Classification of Tumours, No. 3)

[2] World Health Organization (1990) International classification of diseases for
oncology. Geneva

[3] College of American Pathologists (1982) Systematized nomenclature of
medicine. Chicago

a consensus adopted by members of the group, it necessarily represents a view from which some pathologists may wish to dissent. It is
our hope, nonetheless, that in the interests of international coopera-
tion all pathologists will use the classification as put forward. Criti-
cism and suggestions for its improvement will be welcomed; these
should be sent to the World Health Organization, Geneva, Switzer-
land.

The publications in the series *International Histological Classification of Tumours* are not intended to serve as textbooks, but rather
to promote the adoption of a uniform terminology that will facilitate
communication among cancer workers. For this reason, the literature
references have intentionally been omitted and readers should refer
to standard works for bibliographies.

Contents

Introduction

The first edition of *Histological Typing of Soft Tissue Tumours,* published in 1969, represented a major step in the standardization of nomenclature in this specialty area. Accompanied by a glass slide set of more than a hundred common and exotic tumours, this book resulted in the rapid assimilation of a universal set of guidelines and diagnostic definitions by pathologists in many countries. In the intervening two decades numerous changes have occurred, and our committee has been challenged by the desire to incorporate new and exciting findings from the areas of immunohistochemistry and molecular biology into the classification with the need to develop a simple reproducible classification for practising pathologists. The current system, while based principally on standard microscopic observations, acknowledges and cites the use of diagnostically valuable ancillary techniques.

Changes in the Classification

Although the original classification utilized the concept of "histogenesis" or tissue of origin in defining tumours, we have departed from that point of view, acknowledging the impossibility of determining histogenesis by morphologic means alone. This classification is based on the "line of differentiation", or stated simply, by comparing tumours to the normal cell they most closely resemble without necessarily implying origin therefrom. As in the old classification we have interpreted the term "tumours" in the broadest sense of the word and have, therefore, included neoplastic and non-neoplastic conditions.

Substantial revisions in several major diagnostic categories were necessary to accommodate the wealth of new information. The category of fibrohistiocytic neoplasia, non-existent in the original classification, figures prominently in the revised classification even though this group of lesions, ranging from the benign fibrous histiocytoma to the aggressive malignant fibrous histiocytoma of deep soft tissue, still invites debate as to its line of differentiation. Although most evidence suggests that the cells within malignant fibrous histiocytoma phenotypically resemble fibroblasts, it seems pointless to change a well-accepted, albeit imperfect, term that interferes little with diagnostic practices. Among the fibroblastic tumours, the term "fibromatosis", formerly used very loosely to refer to a variety of lesions ranging from benign reactive lesions (keloid) to rather aggressive neoplastic ones (extra-abdominal desmoid tumour), refers to a histologically homogeneous family of lesions that varies in its local recurrence rate but that uniformly does not metastasize. Although one will note few apparent changes in the classification of lipomatous tumours, a significant terminologic change has been suggested with the substitution of "atypical lipoma" for "well-differentiated liposarcomas of superficial soft tissue" on the ground that these lesions seldom recur. Retention of the term "well-differentiated liposarcoma" for similar tumours in deep soft tissues of the extremity and in body cavities has been endorsed to reflect the high recurrence rate of such lesions in both locations and the mortality associated with those in the latter. The entity of dedifferentiated liposarcoma was added because of the growing appreciation that differentiated lipomatous tumours, like some bone tumours (e.g. well-differentiated chondrosarcoma), can, with time, progress to higher grade lesions with metastatic potential. A category of borderline or intermediate vascular tumours (haemangioendothelioma) was created for three newly described entities which require separation from angiosarcoma (epithelioid haemangioendothelioma, spindle cell haemangioendothelioma and endovascular papillary angioendothelioma). Mesothelial tumours, too, have been expanded by the addition of three benign tumours (fibrous mesothelioma, multicystic mesothelioma, well-differentiated papillary mesothelioma). Our panel is particularly indebted to the Intergroup Rhabdomyosarcoma Study, which shared its collective experience with this group in revising the classification of rhabdomyosarcoma. Through this exchange it was our hope of reaching a common classification for this group of childhood tumours. Finally, this classification adds over 40 newly described entities to the old classification including myofibromatosis, giant cell fibroblastoma, plexifom fibrous histiocytoma, angiomatoid fibrous histiocytoma, angiomyxoma, parachordoma, ossifying fibromyxoid tumour, epithelioid sarcoma, extraskeletal Ewing sarcoma, malignant rhabdoid tumour, spindle cell rhabdomyosarcoma and desmoplastic small cell tumour of children and young adults.

Evaluation of Soft Tissue Tumours

The vast majority of soft tissue tumours require biopsy prior to definitive therapy. Thus the pathologist plays a central role in the evaluation of these tumours and it is his/her responsibility to assess the adequacy of the diagnostic biopsy. Except for very small superficial lesions that are amenable to excisional biopsy, most soft tissue lesions require an incisional biopsy. Although needle biopsies are used with increasing frequency, they are best interpreted by pathologists, experienced with this technique, who work closely with a multidisciplinary team of clinicians. Needle biopsy may be used more routinely in documenting recurrent or metastatic disease once a primary diagnosis has been established, however. Whether a frozen section is performed at the time of biopsy depends on whether immediate intra-operative therapeutic action will be taken. In most centres definitive surgery awaits the results of a permanent section diagnosis so that frozen section is used principally to confirm that viable or representative tissue has been obtained.

Grading and Staging of Sarcomas

Once the diagnosis of a sarcoma has been established, the single most important piece of information with which the pathologist can provide the clinician is the grade of the lesion. Unfortunately, to date there is no grading system which has been accepted worldwide. Although it was not the task of this panel to either formulate or endorse a specific system, we wish to encourage the practice of grading sarcomas using whatever regional system that has been devised and systematically validated. Most grading systems presuppose an accurate histological diagnosis (Tables 1–3), and some even a priori assign a grade to certain types of sarcomas. For example, in the system proposed by Costa et al. (Table 2) the diagnosis of a well-differentiated liposarcoma automatically receives a grade of I and requires no additional analysis of features. In the system devised by Myre Jensen et al. (Table 3) all embryonal and alveolar rhabdomyosarcomas, synovial sarcoma and malignant schwannoma are considered grade III. All major grading systems utilize pleomorphism, mitotic rate and necrosis in analyzing sarcomas, but differ in the weight accorded to these factors in arriving at the final grade and in the number

Table 1. French Federation of Cancer Centres: histopathological grading of soft tissue sarcomas[1]

Tumour differentiation

    Score 1: sarcomas closely resemble normal adult tissue, for example, well-differentiated liposarcoma

    Score 2: sarcomas for which histological typing is certain, for example, biphasic synovial sarcoma

    Score 3: embryonal sarcomas, undifferentiated sarcomas and sarcomas of doubtful tumour type

Mitosis count	Tumour necrosis
Score 1: 0 to 9/10 fields[a]	Score 0: no necrosis on any slide
Score 2: 10 to 19/10 fields	Score 1: less than 50 % tumour necrosis
Score 3: more than 20/10 fields	Score 2: more than 50 % tumour necrosis
	Grade 1: score 2–3
	Grade 2: score 4–5
	Grade 3: score 6–8

[a] A field measured 0.1734 mm².

Table 2. National Cancer Institute (USA): histopathological grading of soft tissue sarcomas[2]

Grade I	Grade II–III[a]
Well-differentiated liposarcoma	Round cell liposarcoma
Myxoid liposarcoma	Malignant fibrous histiocytoma
Dermatofibrosarcoma protuberans	Clear cell sarcoma
	Angiosarcoma
Grade I–III	Epithelioid sarcoma
Leiomyosarcoma	Malignant granular cell tumour
Chondrosarcoma	Fibrosarcoma
Malignant peripheral nerve sheath tumour	**Grade III**
Haemangiopericytoma	Ewing sarcoma
	Rhabdomyosarcoma
	Osteosarcoma
	Alveolar sort part sarcoma
	Synovial sarcoma

[a] Distinction between grade II and III lesions is based primarily on necrosis. Grade II is defined as no or minimal (< 15 %) necrosis whereas grade III is moderate or marked (> 15 %) necrosis.

of designated grades. The overall trend is to employ three grades,[1,2,4] although Markhede et al.[3] endorse the use of four grades on the grounds that there are statistically significant differences in survival between grade III and IV patients. Despite these differences each has been shown to correlate with survival or to predict outcome, so that it may not matter

Table 3. Centre for Bone and Soft Tissue Tumours Aarhus, Denmark[4]: histopathological grading of soft tissue tumours

A:	Number of mitoses/10 HPF (2.5 mm^2)
B:	Mean score (1, 2, 3) based on a semiquantitative evaluation of cellularity (relative to stroma), anaplasia, necrobiosis
Grade I:	< 1 mitosis/10 HPF (mean score B = 1)
Grade II:	< 1 mitosis/10 HPF (mean score B = 2,3) or 1–5 mitosis/10 HPF (mean score B = 1 or 2)
Grade III:	1–5 mitoses/10 HPF (mean score B = 3) or > 5 mitoses/10 HPF (mean score B = 1, 2, 3)

HPF, high-power field.

Table 4. Staging of sarcomas: TNM classification[5,6]

T:		Primary tumour
	TX	Primary tumour cannot be assessed
	T0	No evidence of primary tumour
	T1	Tumour 5 cm or less in greatest dimension
	T2	Tumour more than 5 cm in greatest dimension
N:		Regional lymph nodes
	NX	Regional lymph node cannot be assessed
	N0	No regional lymph node metastasis
	N1	Regional lymph node metastasis
M:		Distant metastasis
	MX	Presence of distant metastasis cannot be assessed
	M0	No distant metastasis
	M1	Distant metastasis
G:		Histopathological grading[a]
	GX	Grade of differentiation cannot be assessed
	G1	Well-differentiated
	G2	Moderately differentiated
	G3–4	Poorly differentiated/undifferentiated

[a] After the histological type has been determined, the tumour should be graded according to the accepted criteria including cellularity, cellular pleomorphism, mitotic activity and necrosis. The amount of intercellular substance such as collagen or mucoid material should be considered as a favourable factor in assessing the grade.

which system one chooses so long as one applies the recommended guidelines in a stringent and consistent fashion.

Like grading systems, there have been many proposed staging systems. The most widely used staging system, TNM, proposed by the International Union Against Cancer and the American Joint Committee

Table 5. Staging of sarcomas: stage grouping

Stage	G	T	N	M
Stage I A	G 1	T 1	N 0	M 0
Stage I B	G 1	T 2	N 0	M 0
Stage II A	G 2	T 1	N 0	M 0
Stage II B	G 2	T 2	N 0	M 0
Stage III A	G 3–4	T 1	N 0	M 0
Stage III B	G 3–4	T 2	N 0	M 0
Stage IV A	Any G	Any T	N 1	M 0
Stage IV B	Any G	Any T	Any N	M 1

See Table 4 for explanation of G, T, N and M.

on Cancer (AJCC) incorporates information about grade, tumour size, lymph node status and metastatic disease in defining stage (Tables 4, 5).[5,6] In this system stage is essentially determined by grade unless the lesion invades regional lymph nodes or has distant metastasis. Thus, grade and stage are intimately related to each other, further emphasizing the necessity of conveying grading information unambiguously to the clinician, whenever possible.

References

1. Coindre JM, Trojani M, Contesso G, et al. (1986) Reproducibility of a histopathologic grading system for adult soft tissue sarcoma. Cancer 58: 306–309
2. Costa J, Wesley RA, Glatstein E, Rosenberg SA (1982) The grading of soft tissue sarcomas: Results of a clinicopathologic correlation in a series of 163 cases. Cancer 53: 530–541
3. Markhede G, Angervall L, Stener B (1982) A multivariate analysis of the prognosis after surgical treatment of malignant soft-tissue tumors. Cancer 49: 1721–1733
4. Myhre-Jensen, Kaae S, Madsen EH, Sneppen O (1983) Histopathological grading in soft-tissue tumours: Relation to survival in 261 surgically treated patients. Acta Path Microbiol Immunol Scand (Sect A) 91: 145–150
5. Hermanek P, Sobin LH (eds) (1992) UICC (International Union Against Cancer): TNM classification of malignant tumours, 4th edn. Springer, Berlin Heidelberg New York
6. Beahrs OH, Henson DE, Hutter RVP, Myers MH (eds) (1992) AJCC (American Joint Committee on Cancer): manual for staging of cancer, 4th edn. Lippincott, Philadelphia

Histological Classification
of Soft Tissue Tumours

---

[a] Morphology code of the International Classification of Diseases for Oncology (ICD-O) and the Systematized Nomenclature of Medicine (SNOMED).

2   Fibrohistiocytic Tumours

2.1	*Benign*	
2.1.1	Fibrous histiocytoma	8830/0
2.1.1.1	Cutaneous histiocytoma (dermatofibroma)	8832/0
2.1.1.2	Deep histiocytoma	
2.1.2	Juvenile xanthogranuloma	55380
2.1.3	Reticulohistiocytoma	
2.1.4	Xanthoma	55300
2.2	*Intermediate*	
2.2.1	Atypical fibroxanthoma	8831/1
2.2.2	Dermatofibrosarcoma protuberans	8832/3
	Pigmented dermatofibrosarcoma protuberans (Bednar tumour)	8833/3
2.2.3	Giant cell fibroblastoma	
2.2.4	Plexiform fibrohistiocytic tumour	
2.2.5	Angiomatoid fibrous histiocytoma	
2.3	*Malignant*	
2.3.1	Malignant fibrous histiocytoma	8830/3
2.3.1.1	Storiform-pleomorphic	
2.3.1.2	Myxoid	
2.3.1.3	Giant cell	
2.3.1.4	Xanthomatous (inflammatory)	

3   Lipomatous Tumours

3.1	*Benign*	
3.1.1	Lipoma	8850/0
3.1.2	Lipoblastoma (fetal lipoma)	8881/0
3.1.3	Lipomatosis	74103
3.1.4	Angiolipoma	8861/0
3.1.5	Spindle cell lipoma	8857/0
	Pleomorphic lipoma	8854/0
3.1.6	Angiomyolipoma	8860/0
3.1.7	Myelolipoma	8870/0
3.1.8	Hibernoma	8880/0
3.1.9	Atypical lipoma	8850/1

8   **Synovial Tumours**

8.1   *Benign*
8.1.1   Tenosynovial giant cell tumour   47830
8.1.1.1   Localized
8.1.1.2   Diffuse (extra-articular pigmented
             villonodular synovitis)

8.2   *Malignant*
8.2.1   Malignant tenosynovial giant cell tumour

9   **Mesothelial Tumours**

9.1   *Benign*
9.1.1   Solitary fibrous tumour of pleura and peritoneum
             (localized fibrous mesothelioma) 8810/0
9.1.2.   Multicystic mesothelioma 9055/0
9.1.3   Adenomatoid tumour 9054/0
9.1.4   Well-differentiated papillary mesothelioma 9052/0

9.2   *Malignant*
9.2.1   Malignant solitary fibrous tumour
             of pleura and peritoneum
             (malignant localized fibrous mesothelioma) 8810/3
9.2.2   Diffuse mesothelioma 9050/3
9.2.2.1   Epithelial 9052/3
9.2.2.2   Spindled (sarcomatoid) 9051/3
9.2.2.3   Biphasic 9053/3

10   **Neural Tumours**

10.1   *Benign*
10.1.1   Traumatic neuroma   49770
10.1.2   Morton neuroma
10.1.3   Neuromuscular hamartoma
10.1.4   Nerve sheath ganglion   33600
10.1.5   Schwannoma (neurilemoma) 9560/0
10.1.5.1   Plexiform schwannoma
10.1.5.2   Cellular schwannoma
10.1.5.3   Degenerated (ancient) schwannoma

12   **Cartilage and Bone Tumours**

12.1   *Benign*
12.1.1   Panniculitis ossificans
12.1.2   Myositis ossificans   73410
12.1.3   Fibrodysplasia (myositis) ossificans progressiva . .   73420
12.1.4   Extraskeletal chondroma 9220/0
              Extraskeletal osteochondroma 9210/0
12.1.5   Extraskeletal osteoma 9180/0

12.2   *Malignant*
12.2.1   Extraskeletal chondrosarcoma 9220/3
12.2.1.1   Well-differentiated chondrosarcoma
12.2.1.2   Myxoid chondrosarcoma
12.2.1.3   Mesenchymal chondrosarcoma
12.2.1.4   Dedifferentiated chondrosarcoma 9240/3
12.2.2   Extraskeletal osteosarcoma 9180/3

13   **Pluripotential Mesenchymal Tumours**

13.1   *Benign*
13.1.1   Mesenchymoma 8990/0

13.2   *Malignant*
13.2.1   Malignant mesenchymoma 8990/3

14   **Miscellaneous Tumours**

14.1   *Benign*
14.1.1   Congenital granular cell tumour   76850
14.1.2   Tumoral calcinosis   55520
14.1.3   Myxoma 8840/0
14.1.3.1   Cutaneous
14.1.3.2   Intramuscular
14.1.4   Angiomyxoma 8841/0
14.1.5   Amyloid tumour   55160
14.1.6   Parachordoma
14.1.7   Ossifying fibromyxoid tumour
14.1.8   Juvenile angiofibroma

15   Unclassified Tumours

Definitions and Explanatory Notes

1 Fibrous Tissue Tumours

1.1 Benign

1.1.1 Fibroma (Fig. 1)

A generic term denoting any localized tumorous collection of collagen associated with sparse numbers of fibroblasts.

Various subtypes having a characteristc location or clinical presentation are recognized. Nuchal fibromas occur in a midline location at the nape of the neck and fibromas of tendon sheath on the digits of the hands and feet.

1.1.2 Keloid (Fig. 2)

A nodular overgrowth of scar tissue occurring within the skin and characterized by interlacing broad bands of homogeneous eosinophilic collagen and fibroblasts.

The lesion usually follows some type of injury and has a predilection for black individuals.

1.1.3 Nodular Fasciitis (Fig. 3)

A reactive, self-limited, nodular fibroblastic proliferation arising on the superficial fascia and growing upward into subcutis, longitudinally along fascia or downward into muscle and characterized by short fascicles of fibroblasts, chronic inflammatory cells and focal myxoid change.

Qualitatively similar lesions may occur in the soft tissues of the scalp in infants (cranial fasciitis) or within or immediately adjacent to vessels (intravascular fasciitis).

1.1.4 Proliferative Fasciitis and Myositis (Figs. 4, 5)

A reactive, self-limited, nodular fibroblastic proliferation of the fascia, subcutis (proliferative fasciitis) or muscle (proliferative myositis) which features ganglion cell-like fibroblasts with copious basophilic cytoplasm and large vesicular nuclei.

1.1.5 Elastofibroma (Figs. 6, 7)

An ill-defined tumour-like lesion made up of thick irregular cords of elastic fibres embedded in an amorphous eosinophilic matrix.

The diagnosis is confirmed by an elastin stain which illustrates increased elastic fibres having a characteristic serrated border and central dense core. These lesions arise on a reactive basis primarily in the soft tissue between the lower scapula and chest wall and occasionally are bilateral.

1.1.6 Fibrous Hamartoma of Infancy (Fig. 8)

A solitary poorly circumscribed lesion characterized by three components: (1) well-organized intersecting fascicles of fibroblasts which circumscribe, (2) loosely textured areas of immature, rounded mesenchymal cells and (3) are associated with lobules of mature fat.

Recurrences are rare.

1.1.7 Myofibromatosis, Solitary and Multicentric (Fig. 9)

A benign self-limited lesion having a distinct biphasic appearance with a peripheral zone consisting of nodules and fascicles of smooth muscle-like cells abutting a central zone of primitive mesenchymal cells arranged in a pericytoma pattern.

Although formerly believed to be a multifocal lesion of infancy that could affect multiple organs (bone, lung, gastrointestinal tract), these lesions are more often solitary. Some cases have been reported in adults. In selected cases, regression has been noted, suggesting a hamartomatous as opposed to a neoplastic process.

1.1.8 Fibromatosis Colli (Fig. 10)

An ill-defined scar-like mass occurring within the sternocleidomastoid muscle of neonates. A disorganized proliferation of fibroblasts sepa-

rates and distorts, but does not destroy, the existing fascicles of skeletal muscle.

In the early stages of development, growth of the lesion results in the symptoms of torticollis (congenital wry neck).

1.1.9 Calcifying Aponeurotic Fibroma (Fig. 11)

A diffusely infiltrating mass made up of infiltrating fascicles of fibroblasts associated with moderate amounts of collagen and focal areas of chondroid metaplasia and calcification.

The tumour primarily affects of volar aspect of the forearm and hand of children and young adults; recurrences are common.

1.1.10 Hyalin Fibromatosis (Fig. 12)

An extremely rare, often familial, disease of unknown aetiology characterized by multiple cutaneous nodules, commonly on the head, composed of immature fibroblasts embedded in a glassy eosinophilic collagen matrix.

Additional manifestations of the disease include hypertrophy of the gums, flexion contracture in the joints and osteolytic bone lesions.

1.2 Fibromatosis (Figs. 13–17)

A differentiated fibroblastic tumour with a biologic behaviour intermediate between the benign fibroblastic tumours and fibrosarcoma, having the capacity of recur locally but not to metastasize.

With few exceptions (e. g. infantile fibromatosis, digital fibromatosis) these lesions are histologically identical and consist of long fascicles of well-differentiated fibroblasts having indistinct cytoplasmic borders, finely stippled nuclear chromatin and few mitotic figures. Interstitial collagen varies in amount, but is usually more abundant than in well-differentiated fibrosarcomas. Fibromatoses are subdivided by location and presentation, features that determine the local recurrence rate.

1.2.1 Superficial Fibromatosis

Fibromatosis arising from the superficial fascia.

1.2.1.1 Palmar and Plantar Fibromatosis

Fibromatoses arising from the palmar and plantar fascia respectively.

They occur primarily in adults, occassionally are bilateral or multifocal and may lead to contracture of the hands (Dupuytren contracture) and rarely feet.

1.2.1.2 Infantile Digital Fibromatosis (Digital Fibroma) (Figs. 13, 14)

A form of fibromatosis occurring exclusively on the digits of children.

Slender intersecting fascicles of fibroblasts containing distinctive eosinophilic cytoplasmic inclusions, which are fuchsinophilic in a Masson trichrome stain, distinguish this form of fibromatosis from the others. Recurrences are common.

1.2.2 Deep Fibromatosis

Fibromatosis arising from deep fascial or soft tissue structures.

1.2.2.1 Abdominal Fibromatosis (Desmoid Tumour)

Fibromatosis arising from the rectus fascia and adjacent muscle.

It occurs principally, but not exclusively, in young women in the peripartum period. A significant percentage of abdominal fibromatoses recur.

1.2.2.2 Extra-abdominal Fibromatosis (Desmoid Tumour) (Figs. 15, 16)

Fibromatosis arising from the fascia and adjacent muscles apart from the abdominal wall.

Most originate in the shoulder, thigh and buttock regions of young adults and have a very high local recurrence rate.

1.2.2.3 Intra-abdominal and Mesenteric Fibromatosis

Fibromatosis arising in a intra-abdominal or mesenteric location.

A small percentage of patients with fibromatosis in this location also have Gardner syndrome.

1.2.2.4 Infantile Fibromatosis (Fig. 17)

Fibromatosis occurring in infancy and assuming one of two histological patterns. The first is indistinguishable from fibromatosis of adults (desmoid type) whereas the second is unique to childhood and is characterized by sheets of short fusiform (immature) fibroblasts embedded in a fine fibrillary collagenous background.

1.3 Malignant

1.3.1 Fibrosarcoma (Figs. 18, 19)

A malignant tumour composed of fascicles of spindled fibroblast-like cells often arranged in a herringbone pattern and associated with a varying degree of nuclear pleomorphism and mitotic activity.

Since other sarcomas, notably malignant schwannoma and monophasic synovial sarcoma, share many features in common with fibrosarcoma, the diagnosis of fibrosarcoma is reserved for those tumours in which no specific form of cellular differentiation is identified either by light or electron microscopy or by immunohistochemistry. Fibrosarcomas with a prominent myxoid matrix have been designated as myxofibrosarcoma and overlap somewhat with myxoid malignant fibrous histiocytoma. Highly pleomorphic sarcomas having a fascicular growth pattern are, by convention, classified as malignant fibrous histiocytoma.

1.3.1.1 Adult Fibrosarcoma

Fibrosarcomas occurring in individuals older than 5 years.

1.3.1.2 Congenital or Infantile Fibrosarcoma

Fibrosarcomas identical to those of adults but occurring in individuals less than 5 years of age.

Most tumours occur during the neonatal period as large masses occupying a significant portion of an extremity. Congenital or infantile fibrosarcomas appear to have a better prognosis than the adult form.

2 Fibrohistiocytic Tumours

2.1 Benign

2.1.1 Fibrous Histiocytoma (Fig. 20)

A localized tumour usually in the dermis and, less frequently, the subcutis made up of varying proportions of fibroblast-like and rounded histiocyte-like cells arranged in short intersecting fascicles. Secondary elements such as siderophages, xanthoma cells, Touton giant cells and lymphocytes occasionally are present.

2.1.1.1 Cutaneous Histiocytoma (Dermatofibroma)

Cutaneous superficial fibrous histiocytomas made up predominantly or exclusively of spindled cells are also known as dermatofibroma.

2.1.1.2 Deep Histocytoma

Benign fibrous histiocytomas of deep soft tissue may have areas resembling a benign haemangiopericytoma.

2.1.2 Juvenile Xanthogranuloma (Fig. 21)

A nodular cutaneous lesion of infancy and childhood characterized by sheets of histiocytes accompanied by a varying number of Touton giant cells and eosinophils.

The lesions may be multifocal but tend to regress with time. Rare cases affect deep soft tissue or parenchymal organs.

2.1.3 Reticulohistiocytoma (Fig. 22)

A cutaneous tumour which features sheets of large, rounded, glassy eosinophilic cells resembling histiocytes, some having multiple nuclei.

The relationship, if any, between reticulohistiocytoma and multicentric reticulohistiocytosis, a systemic disease characterized by a progressive arthritis in association with skin and mucosal lesions, is uncertain.

2.1.4 Xanthoma (Fig. 23)

A localized collection of tissue macrophages containing lipid usually arising in response to alterations in serum lipids.

Xanthomas may develop as small lesions on the skin (eruptive xanthoma) or eyelid (xanthelasma), as larger lesions adjacent to elbow, knee and digits (tuberous xanthoma), within tendons (tendinous xanthoma) or along skin creases (plane xanthoma).

2.2 Intermediate

2.2.1 Atypical Fibroxanthoma (Fig. 24)

A small (usually < 1.5 cm in diameter), primary, pleomorphic spindled cell tumour of skin confined to the dermis or with only minimal extension into subcutaneous tissue and without vascular invasion.

These lesions probably represent the superficial counterpart of the malignant fibrous histiocytoma; they may recur, but rarely metastasize.

2.2.2 Dermatofibrosarcoma Protuberans (Figs. 25–27)

A nodular or multinodular infiltrating tumour of skin and, often, subcutis composed of slender, uniform spindled cells arranged in a cartwheel or storiform pattern. Melanin-bearing dendritic cells may be present in a small number of tumours and have been referred to as pigmented dermatofibrosarcoma protuberans (Bednar tumour, storiform neurofibroma).

The tumour recurs commonly, but rarely metastasizes.

2.2.3 Giant Cell Fibroblastoma (Fig. 28)

A superficial tumour of childhood composed of spindled cells embedded in a fibromyxoid stroma with distinctive multinucleated giant cells lining cleft-like pseudovascular spaces.

The presence of focal areas resembling a dermatofibrosarcoma in some cases suggests this tumour may be a juvenile counterpart of the former lesion. This lesion has a high recurrence rate, but metastases have not been documented.

2.2.4 Plexiform Fibrohistiocytic Tumour (Fig. 29)

An infiltrating superficially located tumour of childhood characterized by multiple nodules of cells resembling mononuclear and multinucleated histiocytes circumscribed by fascicles of well-differentiated fibroblasts resembling a fibromatosis.

The tumour frequently recurs but seldom gives rise to metastases.

2.2.5 Angiomatoid Fibrous Histiocytoma (Figs. 30, 31)

A superficially located tumour of children and young adults composed of sheets of histiocyte-like cells interrupted by cystic hemorrhage and surrounded by a chronic inflammatory infiltrate and often a dense fibrous pseudocapsule.

The tumour commonly recurs but only in exceptional cases gives rise to metastatic disease.

2.3 Malignant

2.3.1 Malignant Fibrous Histiocytoma (Figs. 32–35)

A pleomorphic spindle cell sarcoma usually occurring in adults and displaying no distinct line of differentiation. It typically contains a haphazardly arranged mixture of pleomorphic spindled and giant cells, xanthoma cells and inflammatory cells. A storiform or cartwheel pattern may be seen but is usually focal, if present at all.

Several histological subtypes are recognized.

2.3.1.1 Storiform-Pleomorphic (Fig. 32)

The most common subtype of malignant fibrous histiocytoma ranging in appearance from tumours composed predominantly of plump spindled cells arranged in a storiform pattern to those containing numerous haphazardly arranged pleomorphic cells.

The majority of these tumours are high grade.

2.3.1.2 Myxoid (Fig. 33)

A malignant fibrous histiocytoma in which at least one half of the entire tumour displays a highly vascularized myxoid stroma.

These tumours have a better prognosis than the storiform-pleomorphic subtype.

2.3.1.3 Giant Cell (Fig. 34)

A malignant fibrous histiocytoma containing an abundance of osteoclastic giant cells and occasionally focal osteoid.

These tumours have a prognosis similar to the storiform-pleomorphic subtype. They have been referred to as malignant giant cell tumour of soft parts.

2.3.1.4 Xanthomatous (Inflammatory) (Fig. 35)

A malignant fibrous histiocytoma in which benign and malignant xanthoma cells constitute a significant part of the cellular population of the tumour. Inflammatory cells, either acute or chronic, may also be prominent.

This variant has also been referred to as "inflammatory (malignant) fibrous histiocytoma."

3 Lipomatous Tumours

3.1 Benign

3.1.1 Lipoma (Figs. 36, 37)

A tumour composed exclusively of adipocytes without cellular atypia.

This tumour typically occurs as a demarcated mass in the subcutaneous tissue, but also as a less circumscribed, deeply situated lesion involving muscle (intramuscular and intermuscular lipoma), nerve (perineural lipoma, lipofibromatous hamartoma) or synovium (synovial lipoma). Lipomas occasionally contain other elements such as cartilage, bone and smooth muscle.

3.1.2 Lipoblastoma (Fetal Lipoma) (Figs. 38, 39)

A benign lobulated tumour of childhood resembling fetal fat.

It may present as a localized or diffuse mass (lipoblastomatosis) and has the ability to mature toward a typical (adult type) lipoma with time.

3.1.3 Lipomatosis

A diffusely infiltrating proliferation of mature adipose tissue showing no cellular atypia.

This rare condition occurs more frequently in children and may involve sizable portions of an extremity or the trunk.

3.1.4 Angiolipoma (Fig. 40)

A lipoma in which small capillary-sized vessels containing microthrombi traverse the tumour.

These lesions are often multiple and commonly affect the subcutis of the forearm.

3.1.5 Spindle Cell / Pleomorphic Lipoma (Figs. 41, 42)

A circumscribed, subcutaneous lipomatous tumour occurring chiefly in males on the neck, back and shoulder region and composed of mature fat, thick cords of collagen and spindled cells. In spindle cell lipoma the spindled cells are quite bland and resemble fibroblasts whereas in pleomor-

phic lipoma the cells have more hyperchromatic nuclei and may contain a wreath of peripheral nuclei (floret giant cells).

Spindle cell and pleomorphic lipoma probably represent opposite ends of a common histological spectrum. Both are invariably benign, but since their behaviour, in part, probably reflects their superficial location and circumscription, these diagnoses should not be used for deeply situated or infiltrating lesions having some of the foregoing histological features.

3.1.6 Angiomyolipoma (Fig. 43)

A benign neoplasm or hamartomatous process consisting of a mixture of adipose tissue, thick-walled vessles and smooth muscle elements.

This unencapsulated lesion typically arises from the renal capsule or perirenal soft tissue, but rarely can also involve the soft tissue in or around regional lymph nodes. This lesion may occur sporadically or as part of the tuberous sclerosis complex.

3.1.7 Myelolipoma (Fig. 44)

A rare uni- or bilateral lesion arising from the adrenal or retroperitoneal soft tissue and made up of haematopoietic tissue and mature fat.

It is unassociated with haematopoietic disorders.

3.1.8 Hibernoma (Fig. 45)

A circumscribed tumour usually involving the superficial fat of the shoulder and neck of young adults and made up of finely vacuolated brown fat cells.

3.1.9 Atypical Lipoma

A tumour having the appearance of a well-differentiated liposarcoma but restricted to the subcutaneous tissues of the body.

The use of atypical lipoma is endorsed for superficial well-differentiated liposarcoma because of the minimal morbidity associated with such lesions.

3.2 Malignant

3.2.1 Well-differentiated Liposarcoma

A tumour composed of mature fat cells, occasional atypical hyperchromatic cells and lipoblasts.

Most of these lesions occur in mid- to late adult life either in the deep soft tissues of the extremity or in the body cavities. These tumours have a high rate of local recurrence depending on their location, but essentially never metastasize. A small proportion may progress with time to higher grade lesions (see Dedifferentiated Liposarcomas). The term "atypical lipoma" is recommended for well-differentiated liposarcoma involving the subcutaneous structures (see above). Several subtypes of well-differentiated liposarcoma are recognized.

3.2.1.1 Lipoma-like (Fig. 46)

A well-differentiated liposarcoma containing an abundance of mature fat cells and lipoblasts.

3.2.1.2 Sclerosing (Fig. 47)

A well-differentiated liposarcoma composed of mature fat traversed by dense fibrous bands containing atypical cells. Lipoblasts are typically difficult to identify in this subtype.

3.2.1.3 Inflammatory (Fig. 48)

A well-differentiated liposarcoma of either of the above two types which contains a prominent lymphoplasmacytic infiltrate.

3.2.2 Myxoid Liposarcoma (Fig. 49)

A liposarcoma characterized by bland rounded to fusiform cells set in a highly vascularized myxoid matrix containing lipoblasts.

Myxoid liposarcomas usually occur as extremity lesions in middle-aged individuals. They commonly recur but infrequently metastasize. Less differentiated round cell areas (see below) may occur within myxoid liposarcomas and adversely affect the prognosis. Therefore, only tumours with a minimal round cell component should be designated as pure myxoid liposarcomas.

3.2.3 Round Cell (Poorly Differentiated Myxoid) Liposarcoma
(Fig. 50)

Liposarcomas having the same clinical presentation as myxoid liposarcomas but characterized by an admixture of areas containing primitive round cells. These round cell areas display less lipoblastic differentiation and have a less conspicuous vasculature than myxoid liposarcoma. Tumours having a minor round cell component can be designated as liposarcoma of mixed type (myxoid/round cell) whereas those with a significant round cell component should be considered as round cell (high grade) liposarcomas.

3.2.4 Pleomorphic Liposarcoma (Fig. 51)

A liposarcoma containing a background of pleomorphic spindled and rounded cells and a variable number of pleomorphic lipoblasts.

These tumours may resemble a malignant fibrous histiocytoma except for the presence of pleomorphic lipoblasts.

3.2.5 Dedifferentiated Liposarcoma (Figs. 52, 53)

A liposarcoma containing two separate and distinct patterns, specifically, that of a well-differentiated liposarcoma and that of a non-lipogenic sarcoma resembling either a malignant fibrous histiocytoma or pleomorphic fibrosarcoma.

These two patterns may be seen in different areas of a tumour at a given point in time or, alternatively, may be seen at different points in time in the natural history of the tumour. The behavior of this form of liposarcoma is incompletely defined, but probably depends in part on the amount of dedifferentiation.

4 Smooth Muscle Tumours

4.1 Benign

4.1.1 Leiomyoma (Fig. 54)

A circumscribed benign, often cutaneous, tumour composed of intersecting bundles of mature smooth muscle cells.

Hyalinization, calcification and fatty change may be seen in leiomyomas of deep soft tissue. Dermal leiomyomas are often poorly circumscribed and occasionally multifocal.

4.1.2 Angiomyoma (Fig. 55)

A benign well-circumscribed tumour composed of bundles of smooth muscle containing convoluted thick-walled vessels.

This frequently painful tumour occurs typically in the subcutaneous tissues of the distal extremities.

4.1.3 Epithelioid Leiomyoma (Fig. 56)

A benign tumour composed of rounded or polygonal cells with amphophilic or clear cytoplasm occasionally containing a perinuclear clear zone.

Although presumed myogenic, these tumours often do not express muscle antigens. The common locations include stomach, small intestine, mesentery, omentum and retroperitoneum. Those arising from the gastrointestinal tract have been referred to by some as "gastrointestinal stromal tumour". Criteria for recognition of benign and malignant forms of epithelioid smooth muscle tumour are imprecisely defined but depend principally on mitotic activity and size. Epithelioid areas may be present in otherwise typical leiomyomas.

This tumour has also been known as benign leiomyoblastoma.

4.1.4 Leiomyomatosis Peritonealis Disseminata (Figs. 57, 58)

A smooth muscle or myofibroblastic transformation of the subperitoneal tissues throughout the abdominal cavity resulting in numerous, small, non-invasive peritoneal nodules.

The condition occurs exclusively in women, usually during the childbearing years, and is probably related to changes in hormonal status.

4.2 Malignant

4.2.1 Leiomyosarcoma (Figs. 59, 60)

A malignant smooth muscle tumour composed of elongated eosinophilic cells arranged in intersecting fascicles and containing a varying number of non-striated myofibrils and occasionally displaying a prominent perinu-clear vacuole or clear zone. The parallel arrays of myofibrils can be visu-alized particularly well as linear striations using a trichrome stain. Leiomyosarcoma is distinguished from a leiomyoma by greater size, nu-clear atypia and mitotic activity.

Common sites of origin include the gastrointestinal tract, uterus, retroperitoneal soft tissues, walls of vessels and dermal smooth muscle structures (e.g. arrectores).

4.2.2 Epithelioid Leiomyosarcoma (Fig. 61)

A tumour similar to the epithelioid leiomyoma except that its cells show more atypia and mitotic activity.

In general epithelioid leiomyosarcomas are larger than epithelioid leiomyomas.

This tumour has also been known as malignant leiomyoblastoma.

5 Skeletal Muscle Tumours

5.1 Benign

5.1.1 Rhabdomyoma (Figs. 62–64)

A benign and usually circumscribed tumour consisting of mature skeletal muscle cells.

Rhabdomyomas composed of a uniform population of large, polygo-nal, frequently vacuolated eosinophilic cells with occasional cross stria-tions are classified as the adult type whereas those consisting of a mixture of small mesenchymal cells and spindled skeletal muscle cells are classi-fied as the fetal type. Both tend to occur in the head and neck area. A third form, the genital type, has cells resembling those of both the adult and fetal forms and characteristically presents as a polypoid mass in the vagina and vulva.

5.1.1.1 Adult

5.1.1.2 Genital

5.1.1.3 Fetal

5.2 Malignant

5.2.1 Rhabdomyosarcoma (Fig. 65)

A sarcoma composed of cells showing varying degrees of skeletal muscle differentiation. Its cells range from primitive round ones containing a barely discernible rim of eosinophilic cytoplasm to spindled ones having an elongated tail of eosinophilic cytoplasm (tadpole cells) with cross striations or large polygonal cells with abundant eosinophilic cytoplasm. Recognition of rhabdomyoblastic differentiation in some cases may depend on the identification of muscle specific proteins (e. g. desmin) by immunohistochemistry or thick and thin filaments by electron microscopy.

Significant clinical, pathologic, cytogenetic and behavioural differences warrant separating rhabdomyosarcomas into several subtypes.

5.2.1.1 Embryonal Rhabdomyosarcoma (Fig. 66)

A variant of rhabdomyosarcoma featuring sheets of primitive round cells and differentiating rhabdomyoblasts admixed in various proportions.

It occurs primarily in young children in the region of the head and neck; its behaviour is significantly better than that of the alveolar rhabdomyosarcoma. Some embryonal rhabdomyosarcomas display a loss of heterozygosity at chromosome 11.

5.2.1.2 Botryoid Rhabdomyosarcoma (Fig. 67)

A variant of rhabdomyosarcoma recognized on the basis of its clinical presentation as a submucosal polypoid mass usually of the vagina or bladder of young children. Its cells are arranged haphazardly within a highly myxoid stroma but are condensed just beneath the mucosal surface in a so-called cambium layer.

The prognosis of this form of rhabdomyosarcoma is generally excellent.

5.2.1.3 Spindle Cell Rhabdomyosarcoma (Fig. 68)

A highly differentiated form of rhabdomyosarcoma consisting of fascicles of elongated spindled cells recapitulating the late myotube stage of myogenesis.

This form of rhabdomyosarcoma is easily mistaken for a well-differentiated leiomyosarcoma or fibrosarcoma. It occurs almost exclusively in the paratesticular and parauterine region and has a uniformly excellent prognosis.

5.2.1.4 Alveolar Rhabdomyosarcoma (Figs. 69–71)

A variant of rhabdomyosarcoma featuring alveolar spaces lined by primitive round cells and occasional eosinophilic giant cells.

The alveolar pattern is the result of central degeneration within solid tumour nests leaving a residual peripheral fringe of viable cells. Tumours showing solid nests and sheets of cells are referred to as the "solid form" of alveolar rhabdomyosarcoma. It is recommended that a rhabdomyosarcoma showing a combination of embryonal and alveolar patterns be classified as the alveolar type. Occurring in older children than the embryonal type, the alveolar type has a poor prognosis. A non-random chromosomal translocation t (2; 13) (q 37; q 14) characterizes this tumour.

5.2.1.5 Pleomorphic Rhabdomyosarcoma (Fig. 72)

A rare form of rhabdomyosarcoma usually occurring in adults composed almost exclusively of large pleomorphic rhabdomyoblasts.

An occasional pleomorphic rhabdomyoblast within an otherwise typical embryonal and alveolar rhabdomyosarcoma does not warrant its classification as a pleomorphic rhabdomyosarcoma.

5.2.2 Rhabdomyosarcoma with Ganglionic Differentiation (Ectomesenchymoma)

A rhabdomyosarcoma, usually of the embryonal type, containing, in addition, mature ganglion cells.

6 Endothelial Tumours of Blood and Lymph Vessels

6.1 Benign

6.1.1 Papillary Endothelial Hyperplasia (Figs. 73, 74)

A reactive, intravascular endothelial proliferation occurring in response to thrombus formation and consisting of papillary tufts lined by differentiated endothelial cells.

6.1.2 Haemangioma

A benign tumour or malformation made up of mature well-formed vessels usually lined by a single layer of endothelium.

6.1.2.1 Capillary Haemangioma (Fig. 75)

A haemangioma consisting predominantly of capillary-sized vessels.

Those occurring in infants and young children (cellular haemangioma of infancy) may be highly cellular, mitotically active and have poorly canalized vessels. Capillary haemangiomas are the predominant form of intramuscular haemangiomas.

6.1.2.2 Cavernous Haemangioma (Fig. 76)

A haemangioma consisting predominantly of large thin-walled vessels.

6.1.2.3 Venous Haemangioma (Fig. 77)

A haemangioma having predominantly thick-walled venous vessels.

6.1.2.4 Epithelioid Haemangioma (Angiolymphoid Hyperplasia, Histiocytoid Haemangioma) (Fig. 78)

A neoplastic or quasi-neoplastic lesion characterized by a proliferation of benign-appearing capillary-sized vessels lined by plump epithelioid (histiocytoid) endothelial cells and usually associated with an inflammatory infiltrate of lymphocytes and eosinophils.

Many of these lesions in soft tissue are closely associated with a large vessel showing mural damage. The lesion described as Kimura disease in the Orient is not related to epithelioid haemangioma.

6.1.2.5 Pyogenic Granuloma (Granulation Tissue Type Haemangioma) (Fig. 79)

A neoplastic or quasi-neoplastic lesion presenting as a polypoid growth on the skin or mucosal surfaces and featuring a lobular proliferation of capillary-sized vessels. Surface ulceration and stromal edema are common secondary features.

Intravascular (intravascular pyogenic granuloma) and deep forms have been described.

6.1.2.6 Acquired Tufted Haemangioma (Angioblastoma) (Figs. 80, 81)

A vascular tumour composed of irregular nodules of capillary-sized vessels growing within the dermis. The vascular nodules project or protrude into vascular spaces giving the impression of intravascular "tufts".

6.1.3 Lymphangioma (Fig. 82)

A benign tumour or tissue malformation made up of cavernous (cavernous lymphangioma) or cystically dilated (cystic lymphangioma, cystic hygroma) lymphatic channels, often accompanied by stromal lymphoid aggregates.

Most lymphangiomas occur in children in the region of the head and neck.

6.1.4 Lymphangiomyoma and Lymphangiomyomatosis
(Figs. 83, 84)

A hamartomatous process in which bundles of plump smooth muscle cells proliferate in and around lymphatic channels of the retroperitoneum and mediastinum. Lymphocytes may be found in association with the smooth muscle proliferation.

Localized lesions are referred to as lymphangiomyoma whereas diffuse lesions, particularly those affecting the lungs, are termed lymphangiomyomatosis. The process occurs exclusively in women.

6.1.5 Angiomatosis and Lymphangiomatosis (Fig. 85)

A diffuse and excessive proliferation of well-formed vascular (angiomatosis) or lymphatic (lymphangiomatosis) channels affecting a large segment of the body in a contiguous fashion, either by vertical extension to involve multiple tissue types (e. g. subcutis, muscle, bone) or by crossing compartments to involve similar tissue types. In some instances the process may be multifocal.

6.2 Intermediate: Haemangioendothelioma

6.2.1 Spindle Cell Haemangioendothelioma (Figs. 86, 87)

A vascular neoplasm of superficial soft tissue consisting of a juxtaposition of cavernous vascular spaces and a bland spindled stroma containing occasional, vacuolated, epithelioid endothelial cells. Organizing thrombi and phleboliths may be present within the cavernous vessels.

The lesions tend to recur and grow in a multifocal fashion, but do not metastasize.

6.2.2 Endovascular Papillary Angioendothelioma (Dabska Tumour) (Fig. 88)

A very rare vascular tumour of skin and subcutis composed of a prolifer-ation of capillary-sized vessels lined by cuboidal or columnar endothelial cells occasionally forming intraluminal tufts. Lymphocytes commonly surround the capillary proliferation.

The tumour chiefly affects children and is capable of regional lymph node metastasis.

6.2.3 Epithelioid Haemangioendothelioma (Figs. 89, 90)

A commonly angiocentric vascular tumour composed of short cords and nests of epithelioid endothelial cells embedded in a myxohyaline matrix.

The tumour has a low rate of local and distant metastasis. Overtly malignant features (i.e. mitotic figures, extreme pleomorphism) within this tumour portend a worse prognosis with a higher metastatic rate. Similar tumours occur within the lung (intravascular bronchio-alveolar tumour) and liver.

6.3 Malignant

6.3.1 Angiosarcoma and Lymphangiosarcoma (Fig. 91)

A sarcoma marked by the formation of irregular, anastomosing vascular channels lined by atypical endothelial cells.

The tumour occurs in four distinctive settings: (1) as a cutaneous tu-mour on the skin of the head in elderly individuals, (2) as a cutaneous tu-mour in long-standing lymphedematous extremities, (3) as a deeply sit-uated mass in the female breast, or rarely (4) as a deep soft tissue mass. The distinction between haemangiosarcoma and lymphangiosarcoma is not reliably made and, hence, the all encompassing term "angiosarco-ma" is preferred.

6.3.2 Kaposi Sarcoma (Figs. 92, 93)

A neoplastic or possibly quasi-neoplastic proliferation of spindled cells arranged in fascicles and separated from one another by slit-like vascular spaces containing erythrocytes. Periodic acid-schiff (PAS)-positive, dia-

stase-resistant hyaline globules, extravasated erythrocytes and hemo-siderin deposits are commonly found.

Although a highly controversial lesion, Kaposi sarcoma is believed by most to be a multifocal vascular neoplasm that occurs in several distinct forms: a chronic endemic form in elderly individuals, typically on the distal lower extremities, marked by waxing and waning of the lesions with time; a lymphadenopathic form in Africa; an AIDS-associated form and a form related to immunosuppression in transplant patients.

7 Perivascular Tumours

7.1 Benign

7.1.1 Benign Haemangiopericytoma (Fig. 94)

A circumscribed tumour of deep soft tissue featuring bland oval or spindled cells immeshed in a reticulin network and arranged around an elaborate gaping vasculature without endothelial proliferation. Perivascular hyalinization is commonly present.

A pericytoma-like vascular pattern may be seen as a secondary pattern in other mesenchymal lesions so that the diagnosis of benign or malignant haemangiopericytoma is one of exclusion.

7.1.2 Glomus tumour (Figs. 95, 96)

A tumour composed of cells resembling the modified smooth muscle cells of the myoarterial glomus. They are round and regular in shape with a rounded nucleus and well-defined cytoplasmic borders.

Typically these painful tumours present in a subungual location. Glomangioma refers to glomus tumours possessing a prominence of cavernous vessels whereas glomangiomyoma refers to those in which some cells acquire smooth muscle features.

7.2 Malignant

7.2.1 Malignant Haemangiopericytoma

A haemangiopericytoma in which overtly malignant features (atypia, high mitotic activity, hemorrhage and necrosis) are identified.

A pericytoma-like vascular pattern may be seen as a secondary pattern in other mesenchymal lesions so that the diagnosis of benign or malignant haemangiopericytoma is one of exclusion.

7.2.2 Malignant Glomus Tumour

A glomus tumour in which the cells show extreme pleomorphism, spindling and mitotic activity.

These tumours are extremely rare and their biologic behavior is not yet defined.

8 Synovial Tumours

8.1 Benign

8.1.1 Tenosynovial Giant Cell Tumour

A tumour composed of rounded mononuclear and osteoclastic giant cells arising within joints and bursa or along tendon sheaths. The tumours commonly contain xanthoma cells, lymphocytes and hemosiderin.

8.1.1.1 Localized (Fig. 97)

A tenosynovial giant cell tumour growing as one or a few circumscribed discrete masses.

Such lesions usually develop from the tendon sheath of the digits.

8.1.1.2 Diffuse (Extra-articular Pigmented Villonodular Synovitis)

A tenosynovial giant cell tumour growing as one or more diffuse or infiltrative masses.

Such lesions usually arise from the bursa or joint spaces near large weight-bearing joints (e. g. knee) and may have a villous or villonodular growth pattern. Alternative terms are "extra-articular pigmented villonodular synovitis" and "pigmented villonodular bursitis."

8.2 Malignant

8.2.1 Malignant Tenosynovial Giant Cell Tumour

An extremely rare tumour composed of elements of benign giant cell tumour associated with sarcomatous areas, the latter usually resembling a giant cell form of malignant fibrous histiocytoma.

9 Mesothelial Tumours

9.1 Benign

9.1.1 Solitary Fibrous Tumour of Pleura and Peritoneum (Localized Fibrous Mesothelioma) (Figs. 98, 99)

A localized tumour of parietal or visceral pleura or peritoneum consisting of spindled fibroblastic cells arranged haphazardly around an elaborate pericytoma-like vasculature. Hyalinization is a common secondary feature of these tumours.

The tumour is considered one of submesothelial mesenchyme rather than of true mesothelium, as reflected by its lack of cytokeratin expression.

9.1.2 Multicystic Mesothelioma (Fig. 100)

A benign or low grade, often multifocal, tumour occurring primarily in the pelvis of young women and consisting of multiple mesothelial-lined cysts embedded in a myxoid stroma.

This has also been referred to as multilocular peritoneal inclusion cyst.

9.1.3 Adenomatoid Tumour (Fig. 101)

A circumscribed benign tumour composed of small cords, tubules or acini of mesothelial cells.

Common locations include the spermatic cord, epididymis, uterus, fallopian tubes and ovary.

9.1.4 Well-differentiated Papillary Mesothelioma (Fig. 102)

A benign, often multifocal, tumour composed of papillary stalks lined by a layer of well-differentiated mesothelial cells.

Predominantly affecting women, this tumour has an indolent course marked in rare instances by regression.

9.2 Malignant

9.2.1 Malignant Solitary Fibrous Tumour of Pleura and Peritoneum (Malignant Localized Fibrous Mesothelioma)

A localized fibrous mesothelioma in which the histological features including pleomorphism, mitotic actitivy and necrosis warrant a diagnosis of malignancy.

9.2.2 Diffuse Mesothelioma

9.2.2.1 Epithelial (Fig. 103)

A malignant tumour consisting of tubules, acini or sheets of atypical, epithelioid mesothelial cells that grow diffusely and destructively along the pleura or peritoneum.

These are highly malignant tumour that are aetiologically linked to asbestos exposure.

9.2.2.2 Spindled (Sarcomatoid) (Fig. 104)

A tumour similar in its clinical presentation and epidemiologic association to epithelial mesothelioma in which there is such extensive spindling of the cells that the tumour resembles a fibrosarcoma or malignant fibrous histiocytoma.

Some tumours, in addition, show extensive desmoplasia (desmoplastic mesothelioma). The tumour is distinguished from a true sarcoma by focal epithelioid areas and/or by cytokeratin immunoreactivity within the spindled cells.

9.2.2.3 Biphasic

A rare form of mesothelioma in which both an epithelioid and spindled pattern are present and in which there is little blending of the two. These lesions closely resemble a biphasic synovial sarcoma.

10 Neural Tumours

10.1 Benign

10.1.1 Traumatic Neuroma (Fig. 105)

A disorganized non-neoplastic proliferation of nerve fascicles occurring in response to injury or surgery.

10.1.2 Morton Neuroma (Fig. 106)

A reactive process involving the plantar digital nerve that features fibrosis and edema of the nerve and results in paroxysmal pain in the sole of the foot.

10.1.3 Neuromuscular Hamartoma (Fig. 107)

A rare condition in which mature skeletal muscle and nerve are admixed within a common muscle or nerve sheath.

10.1.4 Nerve Sheath Ganglion (Fig. 108)

A degenerative myxoid process involving nerve and presenting clinically as a mass lesion.

It is analogous histologically to an ordinary ganglion cyst.

10.1.5 Schwannoma (Neurilemoma) (Fig. 109)

A localized usually encapsulated tumour of nerve characterized by the juxtaposition of cellular Antoni A areas consisting of short fascicles of parallel-oriented Schwann cells with palisaded nuclei and hypocellular Antoni B areas containing a haphazard array of Schwann cells in a myxoid stroma.

The following represent distinctive variants.

10.1.5.1 Plexiform Schwannoma (Fig. 110)

A schwannoma which grossly or microscopically assumes a multinodular growth pattern.

These lesions are not associated with neurofibromatosis.

10.1.5.2 Cellular Schwannoma (Fig. 111)

A schwannoma made up predominantly or exclusively of Antoni A areas with few or no Verocay bodies. Mitotic figures may be present, but do not adversely affect the prognosis.

10.1.5.3 Degenerated (Ancient) Schwannoma (Fig. 112)

A schwannoma displaying degenerative changes including one or more of the following: marked interstitial or perivascular hyalinization, calcification, extreme nuclear atypia.

Degenerative schwannomas are usually large tumours of long duration located in the retroperitoneum or mediastinum.

10.1.6 Neurofibroma (Fig. 113)

A benign tumour of nerve usually presenting as a fusiform mass and composed of Schwann cells and fibroblasts admixed with dense rope-like bundles of collagen and myxoid stroma.

These lesions occur sporadically as well as part of von Recklinghausen neurofibromatosis. The following distinctive variants are recognized.

10.1.6.1 Diffuse Neurofibroma (Figs. 114, 115)

A variant of neurofibroma presenting as an ill-defined soft tissue mass composed of rounded or slightly spindled Schwann cells set within a fine fibrillary collagenous background. Wagner-Meissner-like bodies are often present.

10.1.6.2 Plexiform Neurofibroma (Figs. 116)

A neurofibroma which extensively involves a nerve converting it into a grossly convoluted mass.

This form of neurofibroma is considered pathognomonic of von Recklinghausen neurofibromatosis.

10.1.6.3 Pacinian Neurofibroma (Fig. 117)

A neurofibroma having small whorled structures resembling pacinian bodies as a prominent feature.

10.1.6.4 Epithelioid Neurofibroma (Fig. 118)

A neurofibroma in which the majority of Schwann cells assume a rounded or polygonal shape.

10.1.7 Granular Cell Tumour (Fig. 119)

A poorly circumscribed tumour consisting of rounded or spindled cells having granular cytoplasm and vesicular nuclei.

The granularity of the cytoplasm is due to the presence of phagolysosomes. Although formerly considered a tumour of uncertain histogenesis, the expression of S 100 protein provides support for neural differentiation.

10.1.8 Melanocytic Schwannoma (Fig. 120)

A circumscribed tumour usually arising from nerves along the midline and consisting of large rounded or spindled Schwann cells with prominent nuclei, and having large amounts of cellular and extracellular melanin pigment. Psammomatous calcifications are commonly present.

The tumour may occur sporadically or as part of the Carney complex (cutaneous and cardiac myxomas, endocrine hyperactivity, spotty pigmentation and myxoid breast lesions).

10.1.9 Neurothekeoma (Nerve Sheath Myxoma) (Figs. 121, 122)

A circumscribed dermal tumour made up of small rounded epithelioid or spindled cells divided into prominent lobules by fibrous septae. The stroma may be focally myxoid.

The tumours usually occur on the upper part of the body of children and adolescents.

10.1.10 Ectopic Meningioma (Fig. 123)

A meningioma occurring in a extracranial location.

In children the lesions are often located in close relationship to suture lines of the skull and have a central cystic cavity. Those in adults resemble ordinary intracranial meningioma.

10.1.11 Ectopic Ependymoma

An ependymoma, usually of the myxopapillary type, occurring in the soft tissue.

Most occur in a subcutaneous location overlying the lower sacrum or coccyx.

10.1.12 Ganglioneuroma (Fig. 124)

A benign tumour with a neurofibrillary background resembling a neurofibroma and relatively mature ganglion cells.

10.1.13 Pigmented Neuroectodermal Tumour of Infancy (Retinal Anlage Tumour, Melanotic Progonoma) (Fig. 125)

A tumour of infancy and childhood usually arising in the jaw and characterized by irregular alveolar spaces lined by melanin-containing epithelial cells and containing clusters of primitive neuroblastic cells.

Although most tumours behave in a benign fashion, a few have produced.metastasis.

10.2 Malignant

10.2.1 Malignant Peripheral Nerve Sheath Tumour (MPNST) (Malignant Schwannoma, Neurofibrosarcoma) (Figs. 126, 127)

A sarcoma usually resembling a fibrosarcoma, composed of spindled cells arranged in fascicles which show varying degrees of schwannian differentiation as evidenced by asymmetric cellular shape, irregular buckled nuclei, nuclear palisading or tactoid structures. Tumours resembling fibrosarcomas or malignant fibrous histiocytomas that arise from a nerve or neurofibroma or that express S100 protein or other neural markers are usually considered by convention to be MPNSTs.

10.2.1.1 MPNST with Rhabdomyosarcoma (Malignant Triton Tumour) (Fig. 128)

An MPNST containing, in addition, rhabdomyoblasts.

10.2.1.2 MPNST with Glandular Differentiation (Fig. 129)

An MPNST containing benign or malignant glands.

10.2.1.3 Epithelioid MPNST (Figs. 130, 131)

A MPNST in which the predominant pattern is that of ill-defined nodules of rounded or polygonal Schwann cells with prominent nuclei and nucleoli arranged in short cords or nests.

The tumours are recognized by the presence of areas of conventional MPNST, by origin from a nerve or neurofibroma or by ancillary electron microscopic or immunohistochemical evidence of schwannian differentiation.

10.2.2 Malignant Granular Cell Tumour

A granular cell tumour having histological evidence of malignancy as evidenced by marked nuclear atypia and mitotic activity.

Malignant granular cell tumours usually show a greater degree of spindling of cells than benign forms and may superficially resemble a fibrosarcoma or leiomyosarcoma.

10.2.3 Clear Cell Sarcoma (Malignant Melanoma of Soft Parts)
(Figs. 132, 133)

A tumour composed of spindled cells with clear or amphophilic cytoplasm and prominent nucleoli which are arranged in fascicles or packets. Multinucleated tumour cells and melanin are commonly present.

The tumours present as deeply situated masses on the distal extremities of adolescents and young adults.

10.2.4 Malignant Melanocytic Schwannoma

A melanocytic schwannoma having marked nuclear pleomorphism and mitotic activity.

10.2.5 Neuroblastoma (Figs. 134, 135)

A tumour arising from the sympathetic chain or adrenal medulla and made up of sheets of primitive neuroblasts forming rosettes and neuropile.

The cells may show partial or early ganglionic differentiation as evidenced by cellular enlargement, vesicular nuclei and cytoplasmic eosinophilia. The tumour is often associated with increased catecholamine production and usually occurs in young children.

10.2.6 Ganglioneuroblastoma (Figs. 136, 137)

A neuroblastoma in which the neoplastic cells have focally matured to ganglion cells.

10.2.7 Neuroepithelioma (Peripheral Neuroectodermal Tumour, Peripheral Neuroblastoma) (Fig. 138)

A tumour arising from peripheral (non-autonomic) nerve and composed of primitive neuroectodermal cells arranged in sheets, cords and occasionally rosettes.

Unlike neuroblastoma, the neuroepithelioma does not display ganglionic differentiation, is rarely associated with increased catecholamine production and occurs in an older patient population. It shares the same t (11; 22) translocation as Ewing sarcoma suggesting a close relationship.

11 Paraganglionic Tumours

11.1 Benign

11.1.1 Paraganglioma (Fig. 139)

A tumour arising from paraganglia and characterized by small, rounded, often epithelioid chief cells arranged in nests or zellballen and surrounded by sustentacular cells and an intricate vasculature. The chief cells contain dense core granules by electron microscopy representing the storage sites of catecholamines and various polypeptide hormones.

11.2 Malignant

11.2.1 Malignant Paraganglioma (Fig. 140)

A paraganglioma with overtly malignant features or one that has produced metastasis.

12 Cartilage and Bone Tumours

12.1 Benign

12.1.1 Panniculitis Ossificans

A reactive bone-producing lesion of the subcutaneous tissue similar in appearance to myositis ossificans.

12.1.2 Myositis Ossificans (Figs. 141, 142)

A reactive and sometimes post-traumatic lesion of muscle in which there is centrifugal differentiation (zonation) from reactive fibroblastic to chondro-osteoblastic mesenchyme.

Typically the center of the lesion is composed of necrotic muscle, hemorrhage and reactive fibroblasts whereas the periphery of the lesion displays maturing bone.

12.1.3 Fibrodysplasia (Myositis) Ossificans Progressiva

An inherited disorder resulting in a progressive, reactive fibroblastic proliferation of muscle, tendons and ligaments with secondary calcification.

In the early stages prior to mineralization, the fibroblastic proliferation resembles a fasciitis. Affected individuals commonly have bone malformations of the digits.

12.1.4 Extraskeletal Chondroma or Osteochondroma (Fig. 143)

A localized tumour usually occurring in the region of the digits composed of nodules of mature hyaline cartilage (chondroma) or bone and cartilage (osteochondroma).

The cartilage may be calcified.

12.1.5 Extraskeletal Osteoma

A localized nodule of mature lamellar bone usually occurring in the region of the digits.

12.2 Malignant

12.2.1 Extraskeletal Chondrosarcoma

A sarcoma of soft tissue in which the tumour cells produce a chondroid matrix as their exclusive form of differentiation.

12.2.1.1 Well-differentiated Chondrosarcoma (Fig. 144)

A chondrosarcoma in which the predominant pattern is that of differentiated nodules of hyaline cartilage having only minimal hypercellularity and/or mitotic activity.

12.2.1.2 Myxoid Chondrosarcoma (Fig. 145)

A chondrosarcoma characterized by short epithelioid cords or trabeculae of eosinophilic chondroblasts embedded in a myxoid matrix of sulfated acid mucins. Areas resembling hyaline cartilage are usually absent in this form of chondrosarcoma.

The majority of these tumours are of low to intermediate grade.

12.2.1.3 Mesenchymal Chondrosarcoma (Fig. 146)

A chondrosarcoma composed of islands of well-differentiated hyaline cartilage juxtaposed to poorly differentiated round cells arranged in a pericytic vascular pattern.

In contrast to well-differentiated and myxoid chondrosarcoma, the mesenchymal chondrosarcoma is a high grade sarcoma.

12.2.1.4 Dedifferentiated Chondrosarcoma (Fig. 147)

A chondrosarcoma composed of well-differentiated hyaline cartilage juxtaposed to poorly differentiated spindled and/or pleomorphic cells resembling either fibrosarcoma or malignant fibrous histiocytoma.

Like mesenchymal chondrosarcoma, this is a high grade sarcoma.

12.2.2 Extraskeletal Osteosarcoma (Fig. 148)

A sarcoma of soft tissue in which the malignant cells produce osteoid with or without cartilage. The cells may vary in appearance from small rounded ones to large bizarre ones that are intricately associated with trabeculae or sheets of osteoid.

13 Pluripotential Mesenchymal Tumours

13.1 Benign

13.1.1 Mesenchymoma

A lesion characterized by two or more distinct, histologically benign, mesenchymal lines of differentiation exclusive of a fibroblastic line of differentiation.

Obvious reactive lesions such as myositis ossificans, which may display osseous and cartilaginous differentiation, should not be classified as benign mesenchymomas.

13.2 Malignant

13.2.1 Malignant Mesenchymoma

A histologically malignant lesion characterized by two or more distinct mesenchymal lines of differentiation exclusive of a fibroblastic line of differentiation.

This designation should be used sparingly and only when other designations do not apply accurately to the lesion. For example, malignant schwannomas with rhabdomyoblastic differentiation are classified, by convention, as malignant schwannomas. It is recommended that when the term "malignant mesenchymoma" is used, it be qualified by the type of elements present.

14 Miscellaneous Tumours

14.1 Benign

14.1.1 Congenital Granular Cell Tumour (Fig. 149)

A benign tumour arising from the gums of infants and composed of nests of cells with granular cytoplasm set in a prominent vasculature.

It differs from ordinary granular cell tumour by the scattered presence of odontogenic epithelium, more elaborate vasculature and lack of

S 100 protein. The absence of this antigen suggests that the tumours are derived from a cell line different from conventional granular cell tumour.

14.1.2 Tumoral Calcinosis (Fig. 150)

A non-neoplastic, but tumorous, lesion featuring amorphous deposits of calcium circumscribed by collections of histiocytes and foreign body giant cells.

14.1.3 Myxoma (Fig. 151)

A benign and probably non-neoplastic lesion of uncertain histogenesis featuring a proliferation of small round or spindled cells set in an abundant hypovascular myxoid stroma of hyaluronic acid containing only scattered, delicate collagen fibers.

14.1.3.1 Cutaneous

A myxoma involving dermis and/or subcutaneous tissues.

Cutaneous myxomas often have a more vascular stroma than those in other sites. They may also contain included epithelial (adnexal) structures. A small percentage are multiple and may be associated with the Carney complex.

14.1.3.2 Intramuscular

A myxoma involving skeletal muscle.

14.1.4 Angiomyxoma (Fig. 152)

A locally aggressive tumour of the pelvic soft tissues, usually occurring in women, that features a proliferation of bland spindled and rounded cells in a myxoid matrix containing numerous large vessels.

14.1.5 Amyloid Tumour (Fig. 153)

A tumorous collection of amyloid typically surrounded by foreign body giant cells.

The association between amyloid tumour of soft tissue and an underlying plasma cell dyscrasia is not completely defined. Amyloid tumours occurring in the absence of a plasma cell dyscrasia are recognized.

14.1.6 Parachordoma (Fig. 154)

A rare, deeply situated, lobulated mass containing rounded vacuolated cells arranged in cords or acini within a hyaluronidase-sensitive myxoid matrix.

These tumours are usually located on the extremities and pursue a benign course.

14.1.7 Ossifying Fibromyxoid Tumour (Fig. 155)

A circumscribed, usually subcutaneous, tumour composed of short cords of bland round to slightly spindled cells situated in a fibromyxoid stroma. The tumours are often surrounded by a shell of mature bone.

Occasional recurrences develop, but metastasis is an exceedingly rare event.

14.1.8 Juvenile Angiofibroma (Fig. 156)

An intranasal tumour occurring exclusively in males and composed of a hypocellular spindled stroma containing an elaborate and ramifying vasculature.

14.1.9 Inflammatory Myofibroblastic Tumour (Inflammatory Fibrosarcoma) (Fig. 157)

A tumour composed of differentiated myofibroblastic spindled cells usually accompanied by numerous plasma cells and/or lymphocytes.

The tumours occur almost exclusively in the abdominal cavity or mediastinum of children. Although the lesions may be associated with local recurrences and systemic symptoms, it is uncertain whether lesions involving multiple sites represent multifocal disease or distant metastasis. For this reason, the lesions have tentatively been termed inflammatory myofibroblastic tumour.

14.2 Malignant

14.2.1 Alveolar Soft Part Sarcoma (Figs. 158, 159)

A malignant tumour of uncertain differentiation characterized by organoid nests of large, polygonal eosinophilic cells set off by an elaborate capillary vasculature. The cells contain PAS-positive diastase-resistant crystalline material within their cytoplasm.

Myo D gene expression has been reported within one tumour, suggesting muscle differentiation.

14.2.2 Epithelioid Sarcoma (Figs. 160, 161)

A malignant tumour of uncertain differentiation composed of nodules and garlands of rounded, glassy eosinophilic cells circumscribing areas of central hyalinization and necrosis. The cells contain cytokeratins.

This tumour characteristically occurs in superficial soft tissues of the distal portions of the extremities of adolescents and young adults.

14.2.3 Extraskeletal Ewing Sarcoma (Figs. 162, 163)

A sarcoma of soft tissue, identical to its osseous analogue, characterized by sheets or vague lobules of primitive round cells having a high nuclear to cytoplasmic ratio, finely dispersed chromatin, inconspicuous nucleoli and ill-defined cytoplasmic borders.

With optimum fixation the cells can be seen to contain large amounts of glycogen. A common non-random chromosomal translocation t; (11; 22) has been identified in Ewing sarcoma of bone and neuroepithelioma, suggesting a close relationship. The cells of Ewing sarcoma also express a characteristic, but not totally specific, surface antigen of the MIC2 gene.

14.2.4 "Synovial" Sarcoma (Figs. 164–167)

A malignant biphasic tumour of soft tissue characterized by epithelial glands situated within a spindled fibrosarcomatous stroma.

Stromal hyalinization and calcification are common. The glands and occasionally the stroma express cytokeratin and epithelial membrane antigen.

14.2.4.1 Monophasic Fibrous Type

A synovial sarcoma composed of an exclusive fibrosarcomatous stroma devoid of glands, but in which epithelial differentiation is inferred by the presence of clusters of round cells with pale cytoplasm and/or the finding of immunoreactive cytokeratin within neoplastic cells. Although monophasic epithelial forms of synovial sarcoma are theoretically acknowledged, there is no consistent means of distinguishing them histologically from a carcinoma.

14.2.5 Malignant (Extrarenal) Rhabdoid Tumour (Figs. 168, 169)

A malignant tumour of uncertain differentiation characterized by sheets and cords of polygonal cells having vesicular nuclei, prominent nucleoli and abundant cytoplasm containing PAS-positive hyaline inclusions (rhabdoid cells).

The hyaline material corresponds to the presence of whorls of intermediate filaments of keratin and vimentin. The uniformity of the cells and the absence of desmin distinguishes this neoplasm from a rhabdomyosarcoma. While originally described in the kidney in children, extrarenal rhabdoid tumours have been described both in children and adults. Rhabdoid cells are occasionally present in other sarcomas.

14.2.6 Desmoplastic Small Cell Tumour of Children and Young Adults (Fig. 170)

A malignant tumour composed of cohesive epithelial-like nests of small round cells surrounded by a prominent desmoplastic stroma.

Although displaying little differentiation by light microscopy, the cells express a number of antigens including keratin, neuron-specific enolase and desmin. The tumour occurs almost exclusively within the abdominal cavity.

15 Unclassified Tumours

Primary benign or malignant soft tissue tumours which cannot be placed into one of the above categories.

Unless otherwise stated, all the preparations shown in the photomicrographs reproduced on the following pages were stained with haematoxylin-eosin.

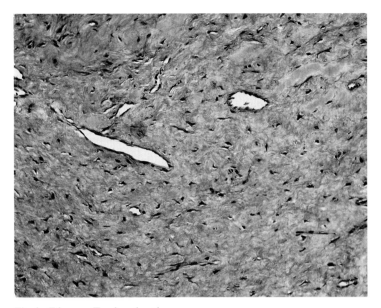

Fig. 1. *Fibroma.* Tendon sheath

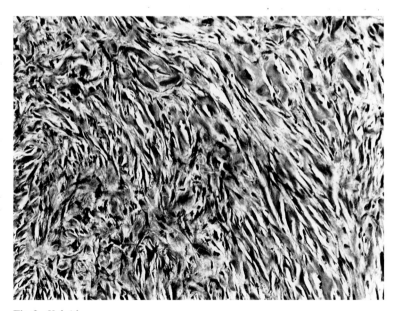

Fig. 2. *Keloid*

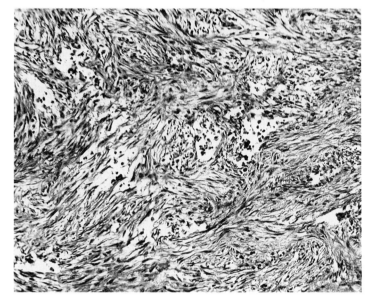

Fig. 3. *Nodular fasciitis*

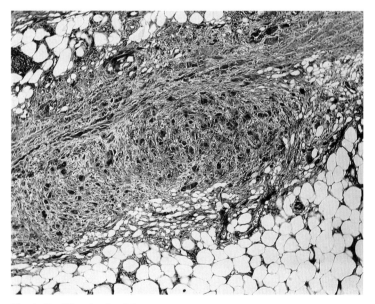

Fig. 4. *Proliferative fasciitis*

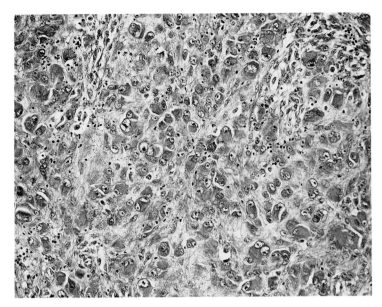

Fig. 5. *Proliferative fasciitis.* Ganglion-like fibroblasts are present

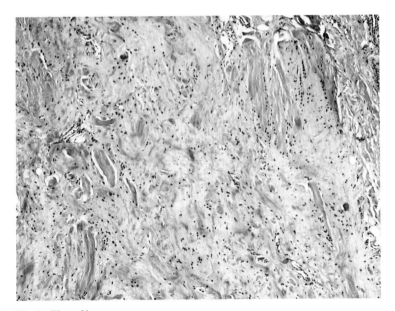

Fig. 6. *Elastofibroma*

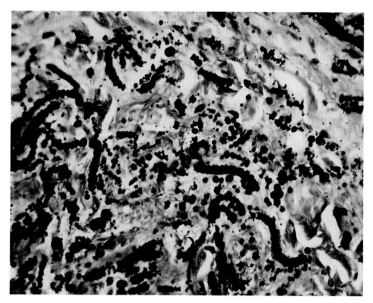

Fig. 7. *Elastofibroma.* Elastinophilic fibers with serrated borders. Elastin stain

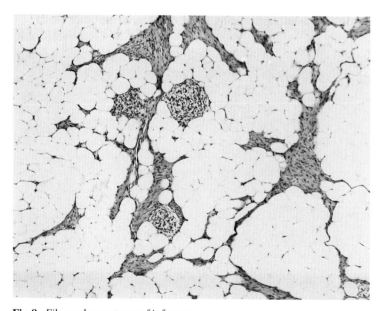

Fig. 8. *Fibrous hamartoma of infancy*

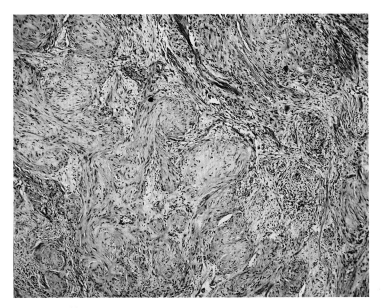

Fig. 9. *Myofibromatosis*

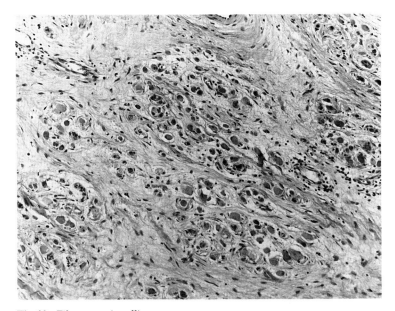

Fig. 10. *Fibromatosis colli*

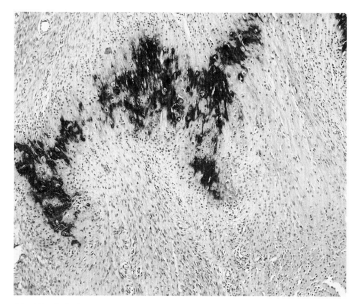

Fig. 11. *Calcifying aponeurotic fibroma*

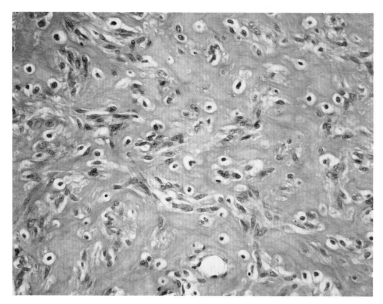

Fig. 12. *Hyalin fibromatosis*

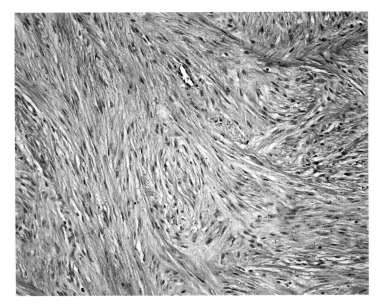

Fig. 13. *Infantile digital fibromatosis*

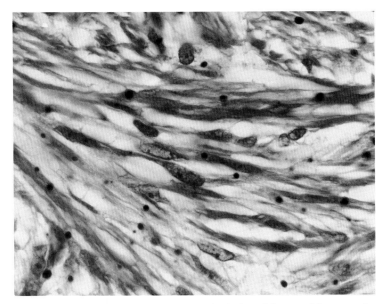

Fig. 14. *Infantile digital fibromatosis.* Cytoplasmic inclusions. Masson trichrome stain

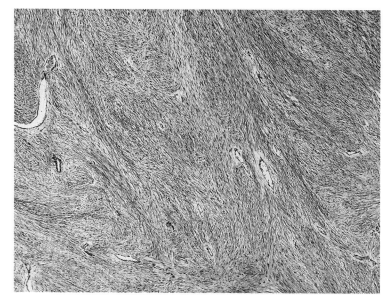

Fig. 15. *Extra-abdominal fibromatosis*

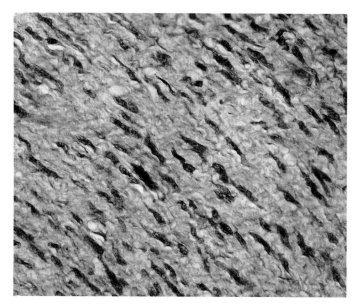

Fig. 16. *Extra-abdominal fibromatosis*

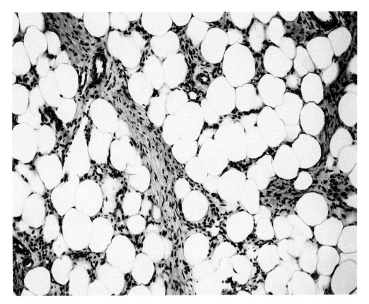

Fig. 17. *Infantile fibromatosis*

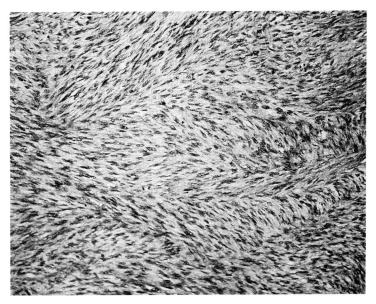

Fig. 18. *Fibrosarcoma* (low grade)

60

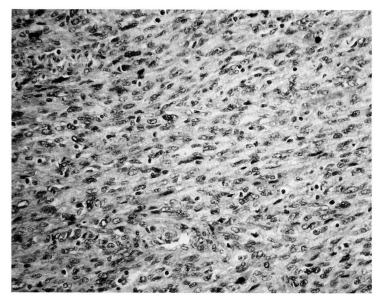

Fig. 19. *Fibrosarcoma* (high grade). Greater cellularity, atypia and mitotic activity than the tumour depicted in Fig. 18. (Reprinted with permission from Am J Surg Pathol 10 (Suppl): 14–25, 1986)

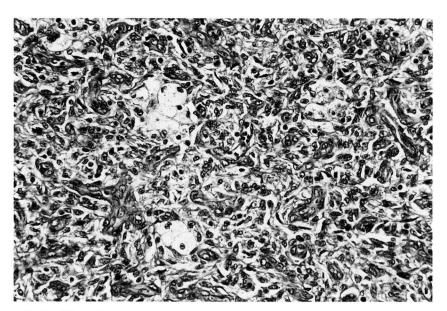

Fig. 20. *Fibrous histiocytoma*

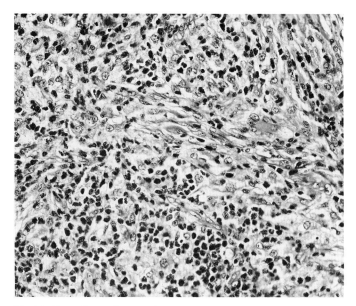

Fig. 21. *Juvenile xanthogranuloma*

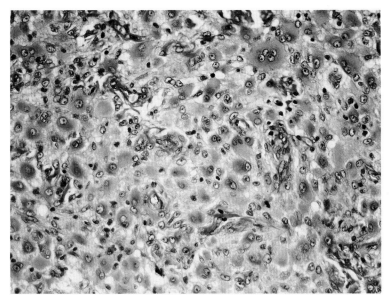

Fig. 22. *Reticulohistiocytoma.* (Reprinted with permission from F. Enzinger and S. W. Weiss, Soft Tissue Tumors, 2nd edn, 1988, Mosby, St. Louis)

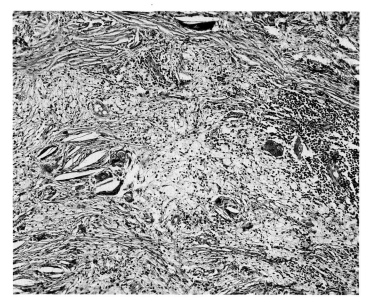

Fig. 23. *Xanthoma.* (Reprinted with permission from F. Enzinger and S. W. Weiss, Soft Tissue Tumors, 2nd edn, 1988, Mosby, St. Louis)

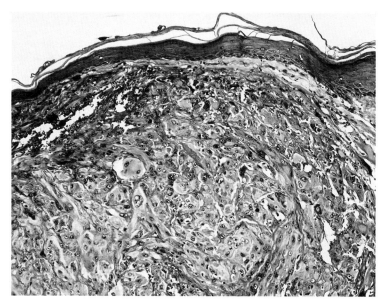

Fig. 24. *Atypical fibroxanthoma*

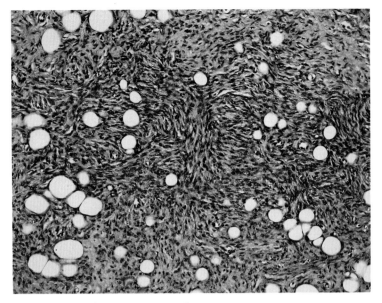

Fig. 25. *Dermatofibrosarcoma protuberans*

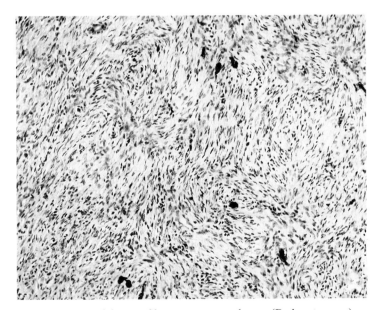

Fig. 26. *Pigmented dermatofibrosarcoma protuberans* (Bednar tumour)

64

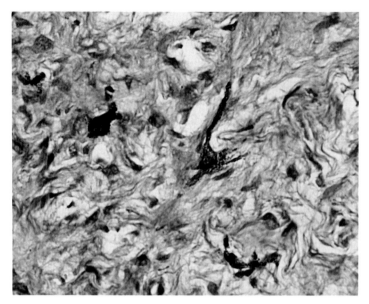

Fig. 27. *Pigmented dermatofibrosarcoma protuberans* (Bednar tumour). Pigmented
dendritic cells

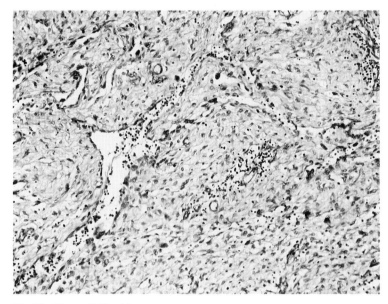

Fig. 28. *Giant cell fibroblastoma*

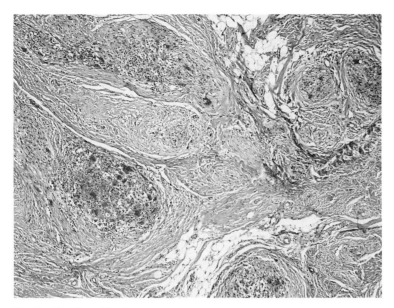

Fig. 29. *Plexiform fibrohistiocytic tumour*

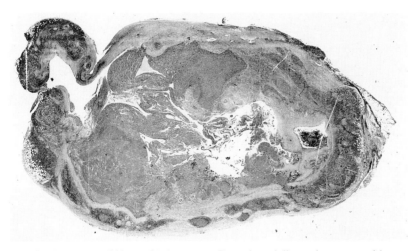

Fig. 30. *Angiomatoid fibrous histiocytoma.* Central partially cystic tumour with surrounding dense fibrous pseudocapsule and inflammatory infiltrate. (Reprinted with permission from Cancer 44: 2147, 1979)

66

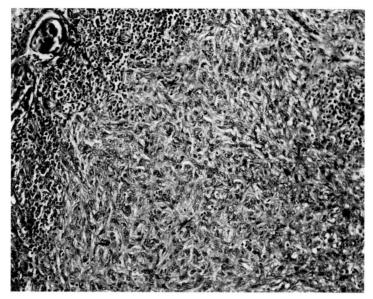

Fig. 31. *Angiomatoid fibrous histiocytoma.* Interface between tumour and inflammatory infiltrate. (Reprinted with permission from Cancer 44: 2147, 1979)

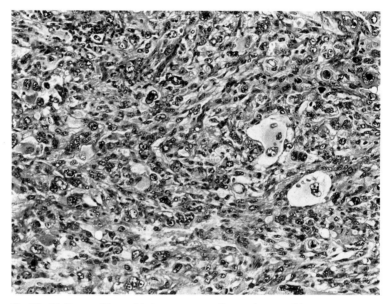

Fig. 32. *Malignant fibrous histiocytoma, storiform-pleomorphic type*

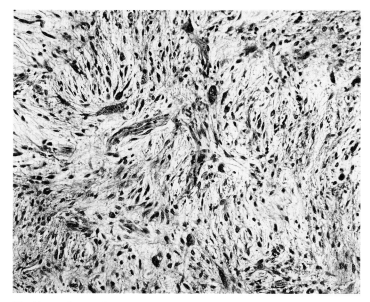

Fig. 33. *Malignant fibrous histiocytoma, myxoid type*

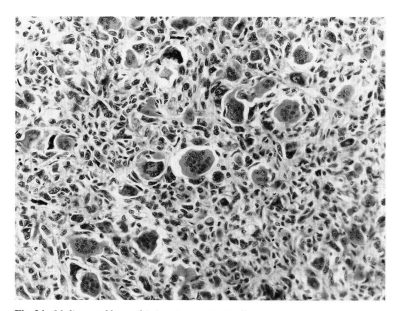

Fig. 34. *Malignant fibrous histiocytoma, giant cell type*

68

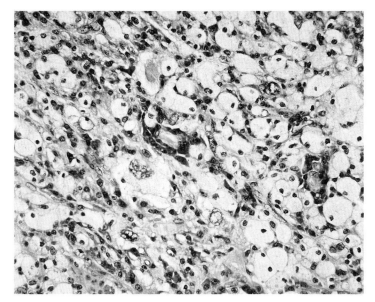

Fig. 35. *Malignant fibrous histiocytoma, xanthomatous type*

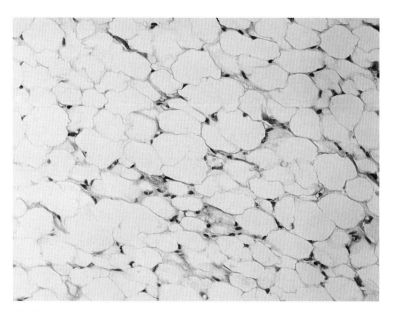

Fig. 36. *Lipoma*

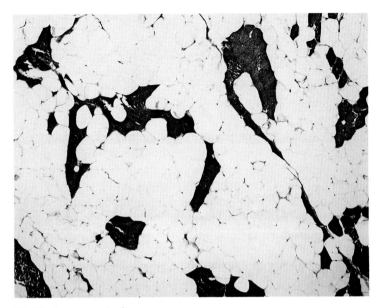

Fig. 37. *Intramuscular lipoma*

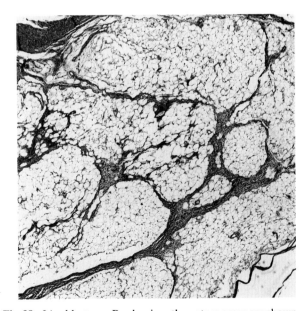

Fig. 38. *Lipoblastoma.* Predominantly mature areas are shown

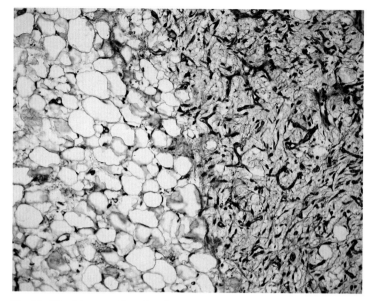

Fig. 39. *Lipoblastoma.* Interface between mature and immature (myxoid) areas

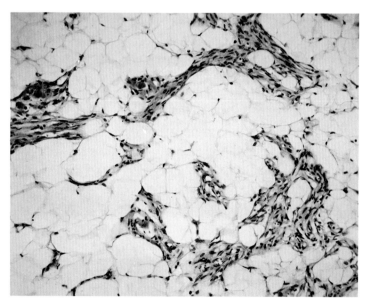

Fig. 40. *Angiolipoma*

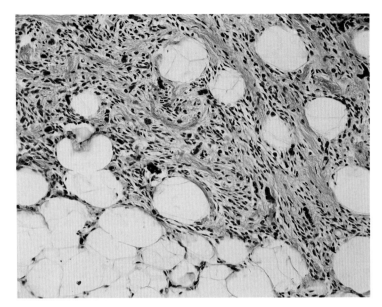

Fig. 41. *Spindle cell lipoma*

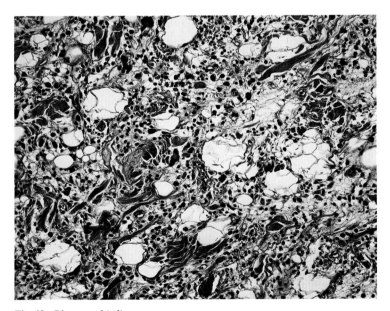

Fig. 42. *Pleomorphic lipoma*

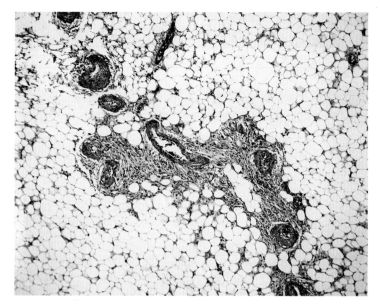

Fig. 43. *Angiomyolipoma*

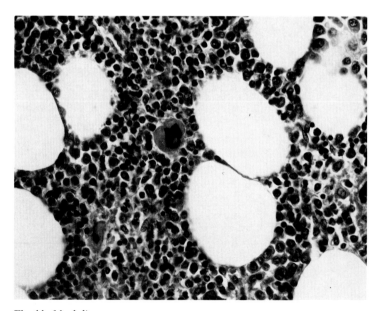

Fig. 44. *Myelolipoma*

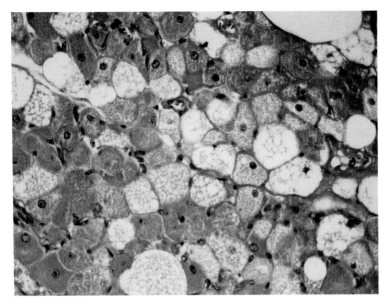

Fig. 45. *Hibernoma*

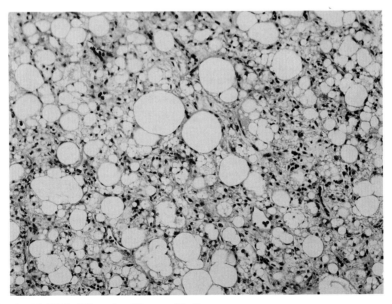

Fig. 46. *Well-differentiated lipoma-like liposarcoma*

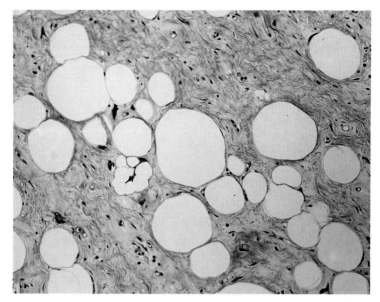

Fig. 47. *Well-differentiated sclerosing liposarcoma*

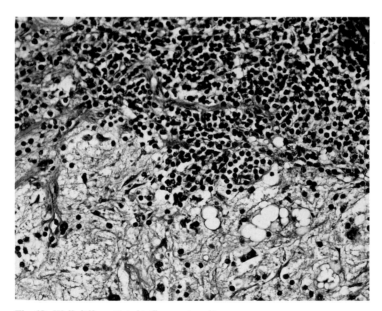

Fig. 48. *Well-differentiated inflammatory liposarcoma*

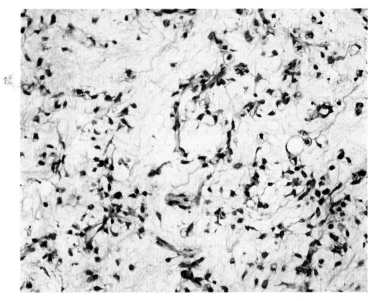

Fig. 49. *Myxoid liposarcoma*

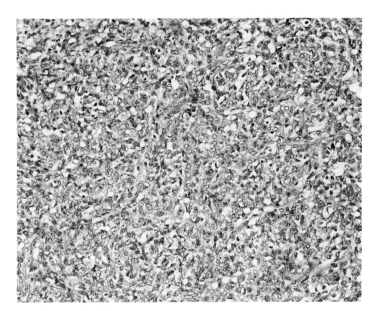

Fig. 50. *Round cell liposarcoma*

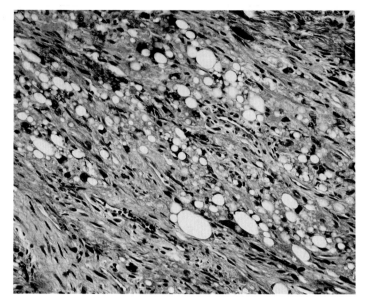

Fig. 51. *Pleomorphic liposarcoma*

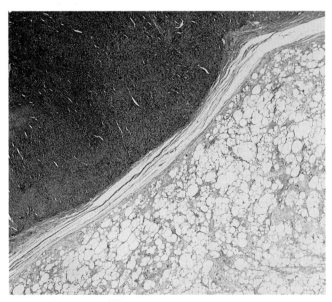

Fig. 52. *Dedifferentiated liposarcoma.* Well-differentiated liposarcomatous component on the *right* and non-lipogenic high grade component on the *left.* (Reprinted with permission from Am J Surg Pathol 16: 1051, 1992)

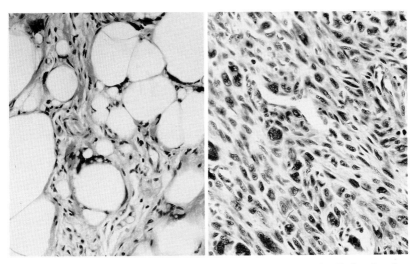

Fig. 53. *Dedifferentiated liposarcoma.* Same case as depicted in Fig. 52 showing the well-differentiated liposarcomatous component *(left)* and the non-lipogenic high grade component *(right)*. (Reprinted with permission from Am J Surg Pathol 16: 1051, 1992)

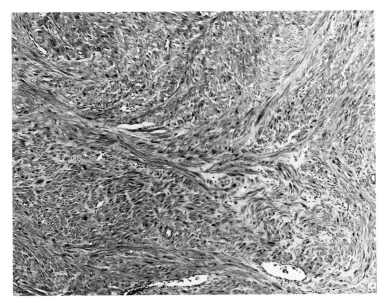

Fig. 54. *Leiomyoma*

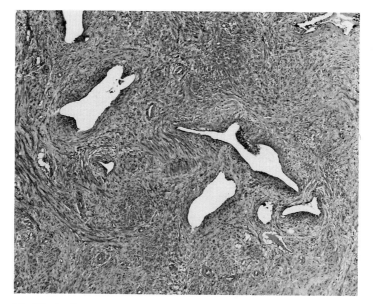

Fig. 55. *Angiomyoma*

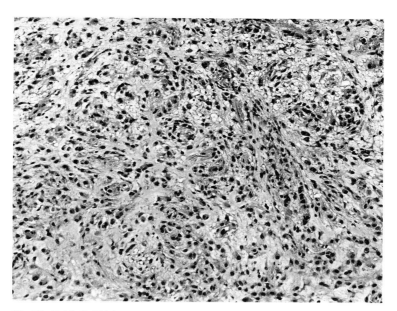

Fig. 56. *Epithelioid leiomyoma*

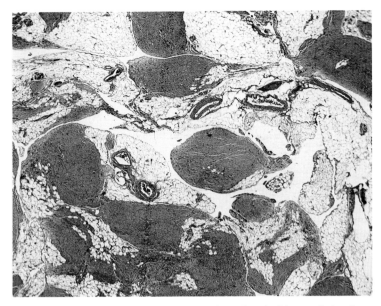

Fig. 57. *Leiomyomatosis peritonealis disseminata.* (Reprinted with permission from F. Enzinger and S. W. Weiss, Soft Tissue Tumors, 2nd edn, 1988, Mosby, St. Louis)

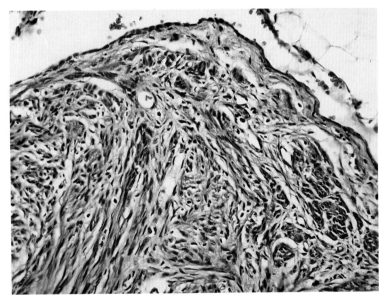

Fig. 58. *Leiomyomatosis peritonealis disseminata.* (Reprinted with permission from F. Enzinger and S. W. Weiss, Soft Tissue Tumors, 2nd edn, 1988, Mosby, St. Louis)

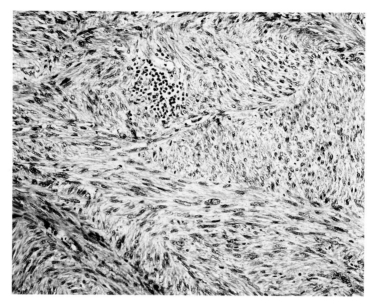

Fig. 59. *Leiomyosarcoma.* (Reprinted with permission from F. Enzinger and S. W. Weiss, Soft Tissue Tumors, 2nd edn, 1988, Mosby, St. Louis)

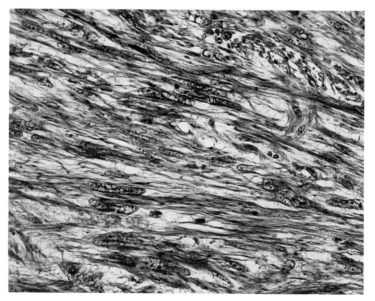

Fig. 60. *Leiomyosarcoma.* Stained with a Masson trichrome stain to demonstrate linear striations. (Reprinted with permission from F. Enzinger and S. W. Weiss, Soft Tissue Tumors, 2nd edn, 1988, Mosby, St. Louis)

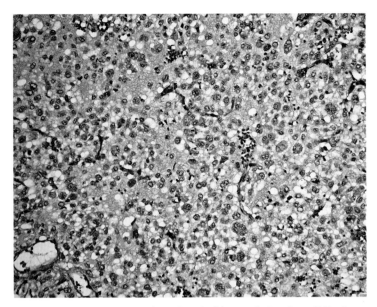

Fig. 61. *Epithelioid leiomyosarcoma.* (Reprinted with permission from F. Enzinger and S. W. Weiss, Soft Tissue Tumors, 2nd edn, 1988, Mosby, St. Louis)

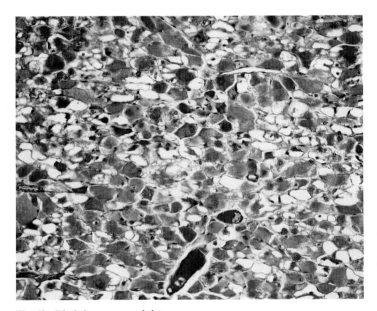

Fig. 62. *Rhabdomyoma, adult type*

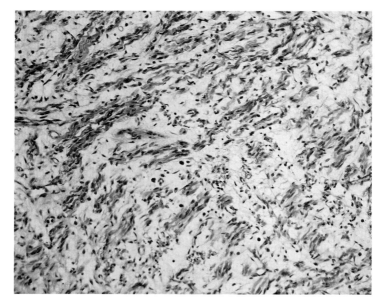

Fig. 63. *Rhabdomyoma, fetal type*

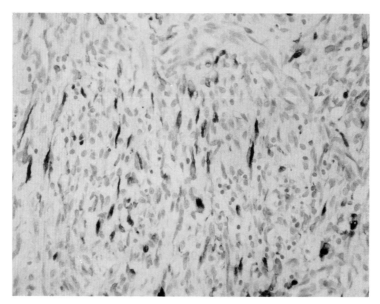

Fig. 64. *Rhabdomyoma, fetal type.* Immunohistochemical reaction for desmin

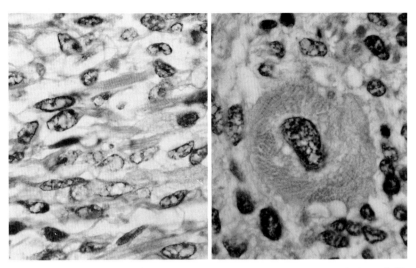

Fig. 65. *Rhabdomyosarcoma.* Spindled rhabdomyoblast with cross striations *(left)* (tadpole cell) and rounded rhabdomyoblast with fibrillar-appearing cytoplasm *(right)*

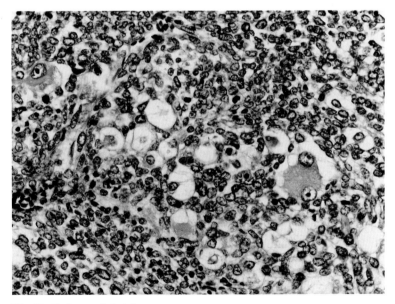

Fig. 66. *Embryonal rhabdomyosarcoma*

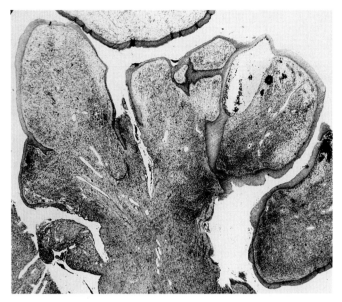

Fig. 67. *Botryoid rhabdomyosarcoma*

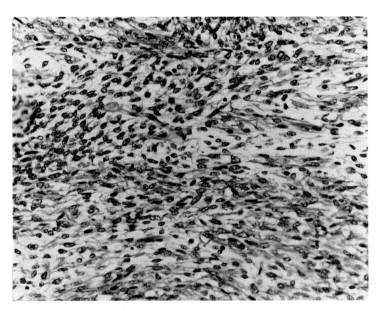

Fig. 68. *Spindle cell rhabdomyosarcoma*

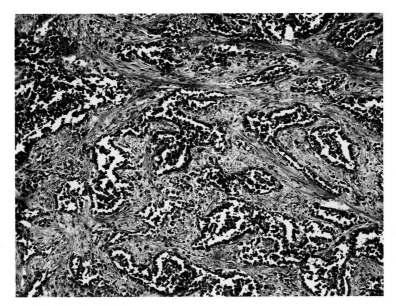

Fig. 69. *Alveolar rhabdomyosarcoma*

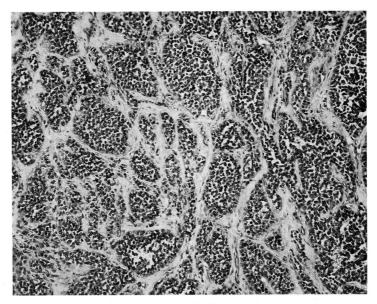

Fig. 70. *Alveolar rhabdomyosarcoma.* Solid form

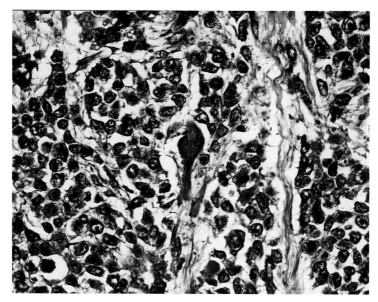

Fig. 71. *Alveolar rhabdomyosarcoma.* Large rhabdomyoblast. Masson trichrome stain

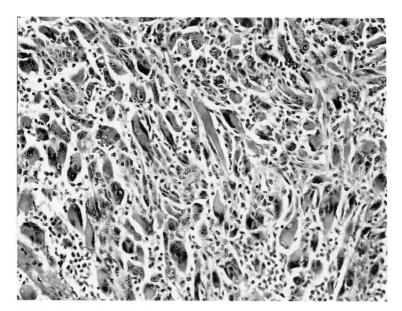

Fig. 72. *Pleomorphic rhabdomyosarcoma*

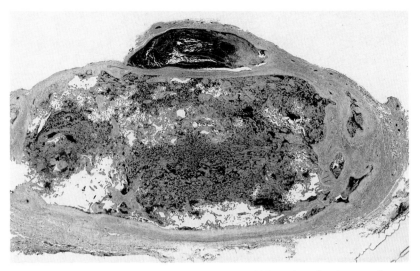

Fig. 73. *Papillary endothelial hyperplasia.* Arising within and confined to vessel

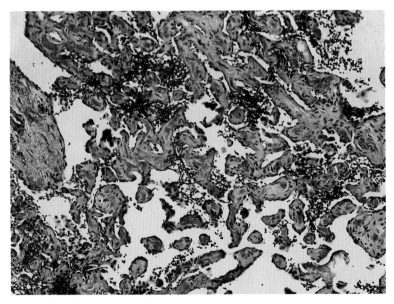

Fig. 74. *Papillary endothelial hyperplasia*

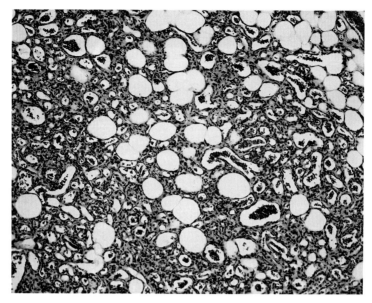

Fig. 75. *Capillary haemangioma.* (Reprinted with permission from F. Enzinger and S. W. Weiss, Soft Tissue Tumors, 2nd edn, 1988, Mosby, St. Louis)

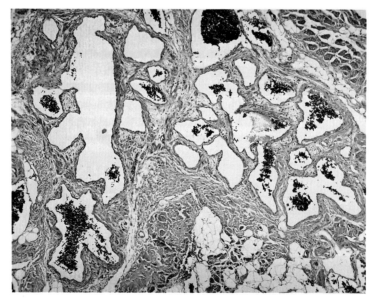

Fig. 76. *Cavernous haemangioma.* (Reprinted with permission from F. Enzinger and S. W. Weiss, Soft Tissue Tumors, 2nd edn, 1988, Mosby, St. Louis)

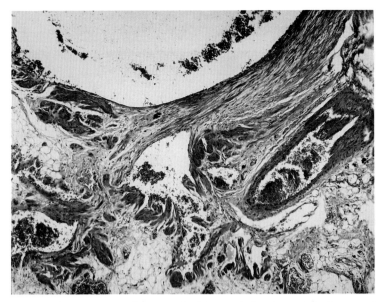

Fig. 77. *Venous haemangioma.* (Reprinted with permission from F. Enzinger and S. W. Weiss, Soft Tissue Tumors, 2nd edn, 1988, Mosby, St. Louis)

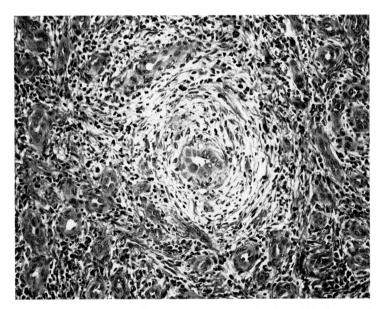

Fig. 78. *Epithelioid haemangioma.* (Reprinted with permission from F. Enzinger and S. W. Weiss, Soft Tissue Tumors, 2nd edn, 1988, Mosby, St. Louis)

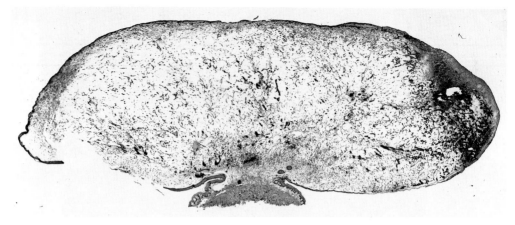

Fig. 79. *Pyogenic granuloma.* (Reprinted with permission from F. Enzinger and S. W. Weiss, Soft Tissue Tumors, 2nd edn, 1988, Mosby, St. Louis)

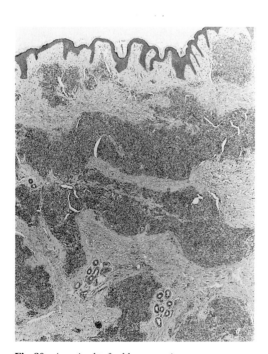

Fig. 80. *Acquired tufted haemangioma*

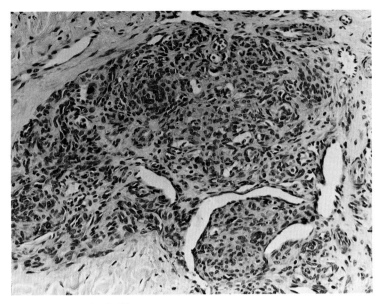

Fig. 81. *Acquired tufted haemangioma*

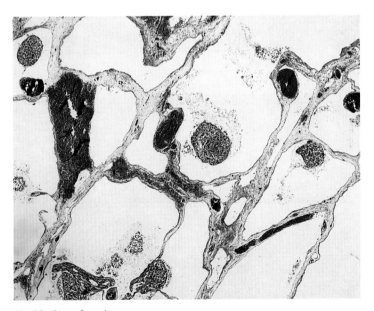

Fig. 82. *Lymphangioma*

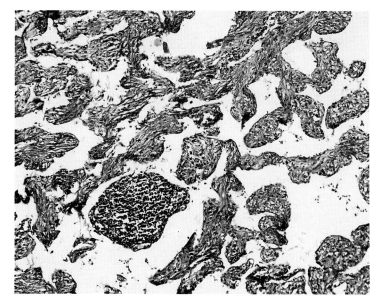

Fig. 83. *Lymphangiomyoma*

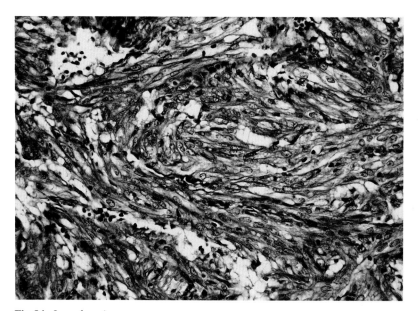

Fig. 84. *Lymphangiomyoma*

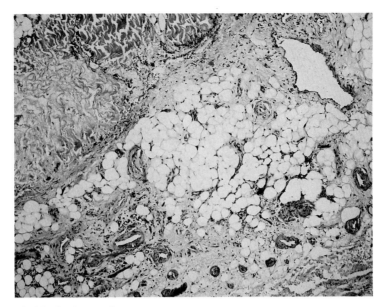

Fig. 85. *Angiomatosis*

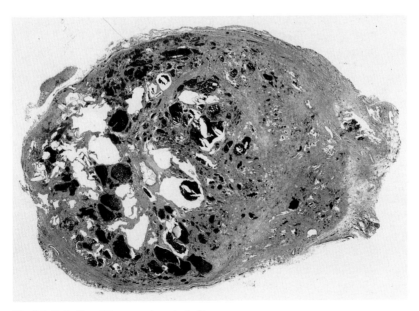

Fig. 86. *Spindle cell haemangioendothelioma*

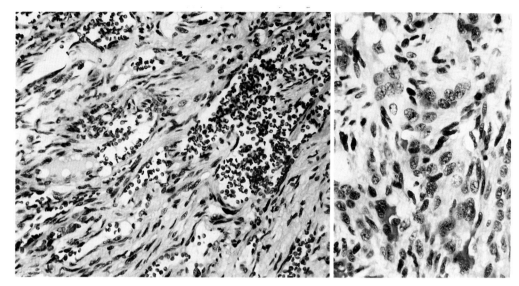

Fig. 87. *Spindle cell haemangioendothelioma*

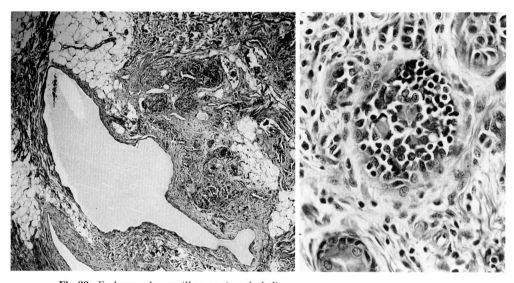

Fig. 88. *Endovascular papillary angioendothelioma*

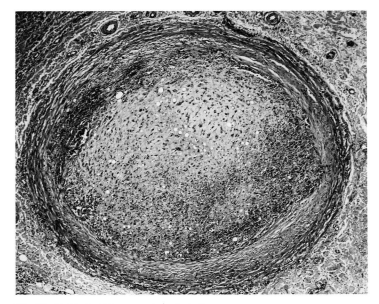

Fig. 89. *Epithelioid haemangioendothelioma*

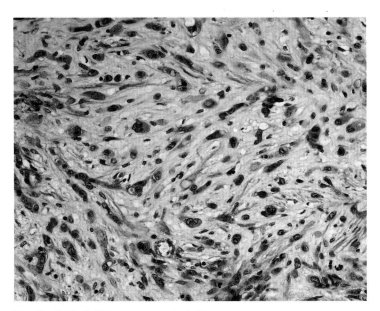

Fig. 90. *Epithelioid haemangioendothelioma*

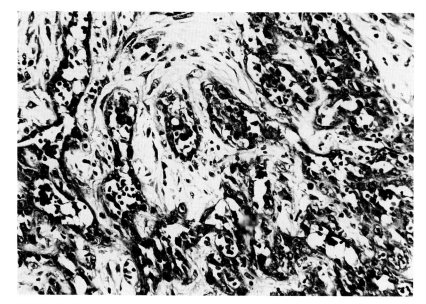

Fig. 91. *Angiosarcoma*

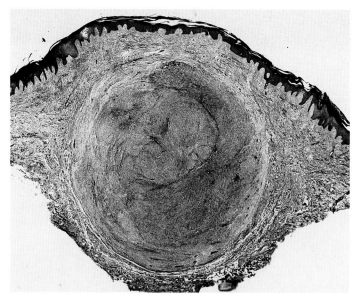

Fig. 92. *Kaposi sarcoma.* (Reprinted with permission from F. Enzinger and S. W. Weiss, Soft Tissue Tumors, 2nd edn, 1988, Mosby, St. Louis)

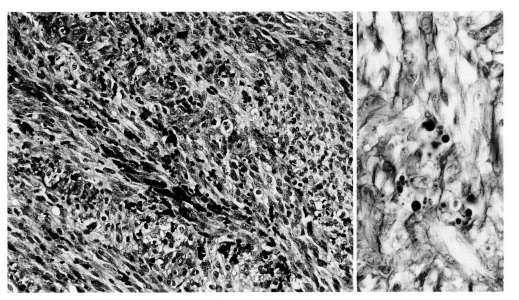

Fig. 93. *Kaposi sarcoma.* Spindled cells surround slit-like vascular spaces *(left)* and periodic acid-Schiff (PAS)-positive diastase-resistant hyaline globules *(right)* (PAS stain). (Reprinted with permission from F. Enzinger and S. W. Weiss, Soft Tissue Tumors, 2nd edn, 1988, Mosby, St. Louis)

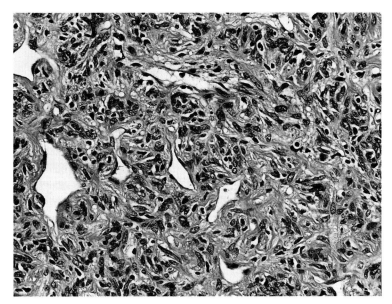

Fig. 94. *Haemangiopericytoma*

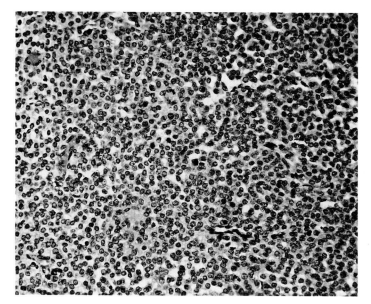

Fig. 95. *Glomus tumour*

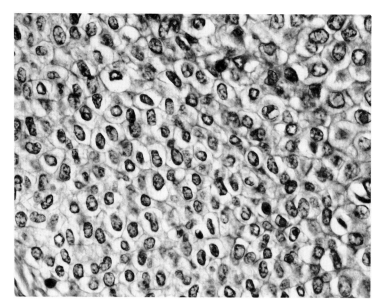

Fig. 96. *Glomus tumour*

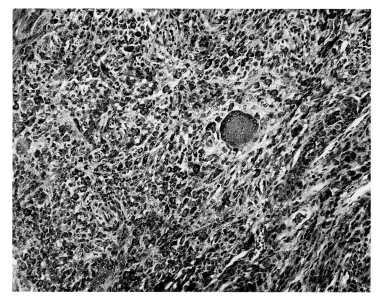

Fig. 97. *Tenosynovial giant cell tumour*

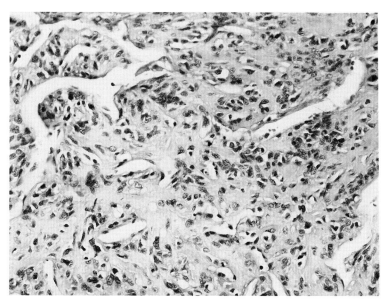

Fig. 98. *Solitary fibrous tumour of pleura and peritoneum*

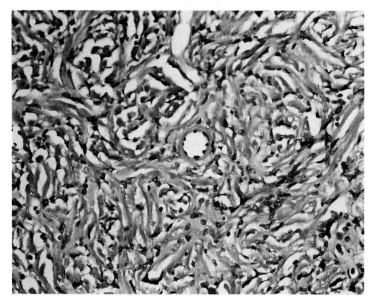

Fig. 99. *Solitary fibrous tumour of pleura and peritoneum*

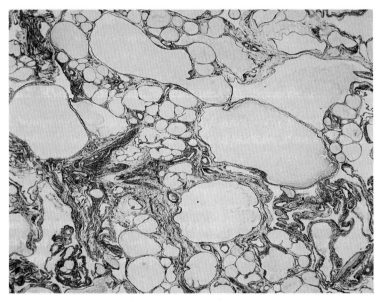

Fig. 100. *Multicystic mesothelioma.* (Reprinted with permission from Amer J Surg Pathol 12: 737, 1988)

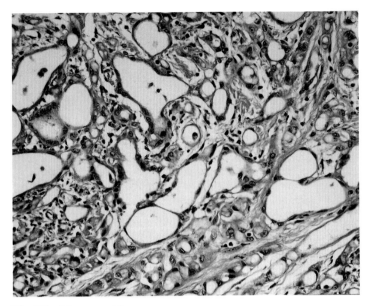

Fig. 101. *Adenomatoid tumour*

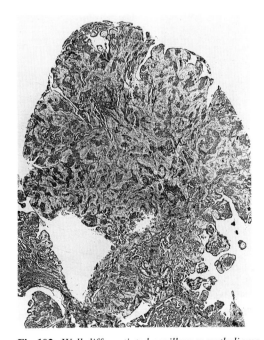

Fig. 102. *Well-differentiated papillary mesothelioma*

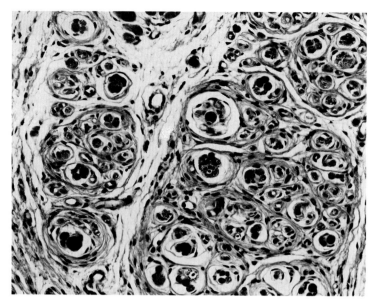

Fig. 107. *Neuromuscular hamartoma.* (Reprinted with permission from F. Enzinger and S. W. Weiss, Soft Tissue Tumors, 2nd edn, 1988, Mosby, St. Louis)

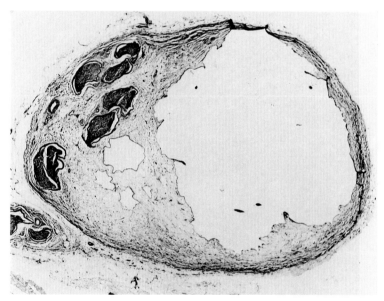

Fig. 108. *Nerve sheath ganglion.* (Reprinted with permission from F. Enzinger and S. W. Weiss, Soft Tissue Tumors, 2nd edn, 1988, Mosby, St. Louis)

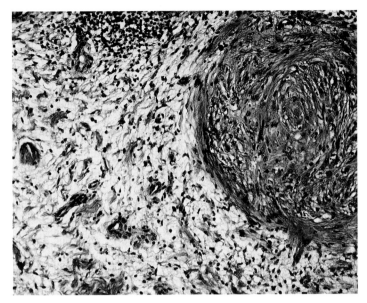

Fig. 109. *Schwannoma (neurilemoma).* (Reprinted with permission from F. Enzinger and S. W. Weiss, Soft Tissue Tumors, 2nd edn, 1988, Mosby, St. Louis)

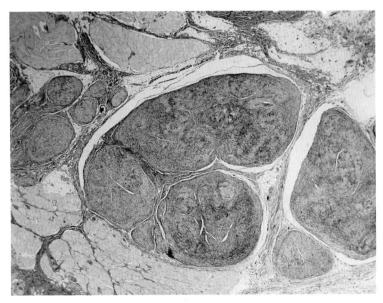

Fig. 110. *Plexiform schwannoma.* (Reprinted with permission from F. Enzinger and S. W. Weiss, Soft Tissue Tumors, 2nd edn, 1988, Mosby, St. Louis)

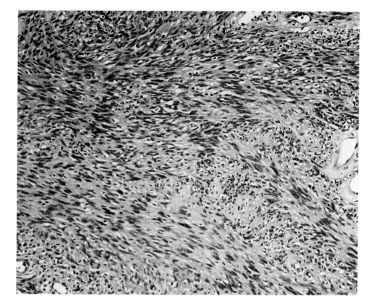

Fig. 111. *Cellular schwannoma*

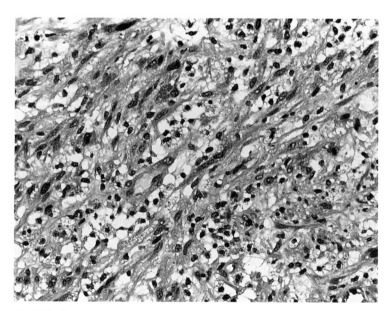

Fig. 112. *Degenerated schwannoma*

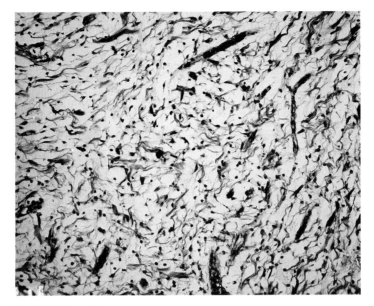

Fig. 113. *Neurofibroma*

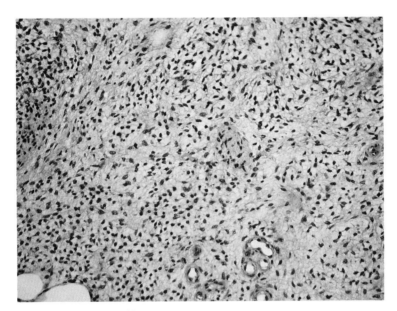

Fig. 114. *Diffuse neurofibroma*

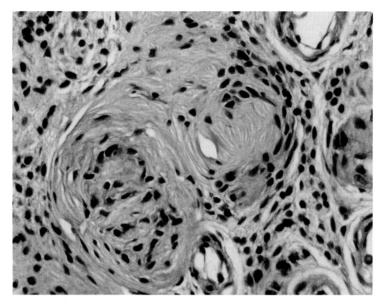

Fig. 115. *Diffuse neurofibroma.* Wagner-Meissner body

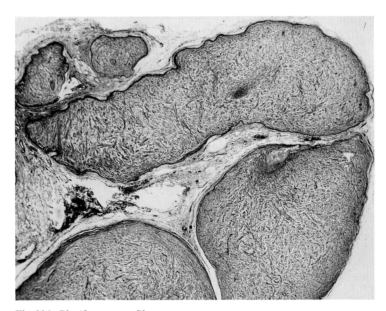

Fig. 116. *Plexiform neurofibroma*

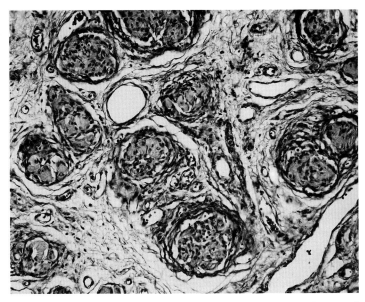

Fig. 117. *Pacinian neurofibroma.* (Reprinted with permission from F. Enzinger and S. W. Weiss, Soft Tissue Tumors, 2nd edn, 1988, Mosby, St. Louis)

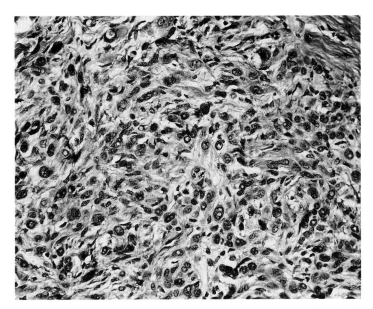

Fig. 118. *Epithelioid neurofibroma.* (Reprinted with permission from F. Enzinger and S. W. Weiss, Soft Tissue Tumors, 2nd edn, 1988, Mosby, St. Louis)

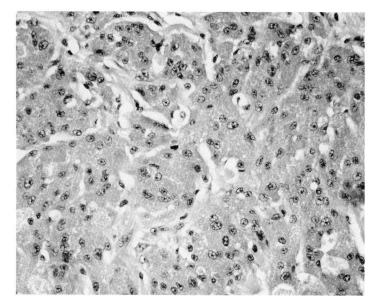

Fig. 119. *Granular cell tumour*

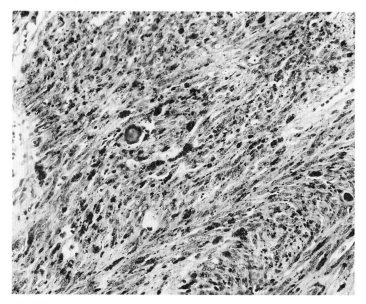

Fig. 120. *Melanocytic schwannoma*

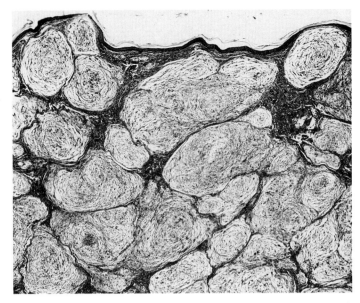

Fig. 121. *Neurothekeoma.* (Reprinted with permission from F. Enzinger and S. W. Weiss, Soft Tissue Tumors, 2nd edn, 1988, Mosby, St. Louis)

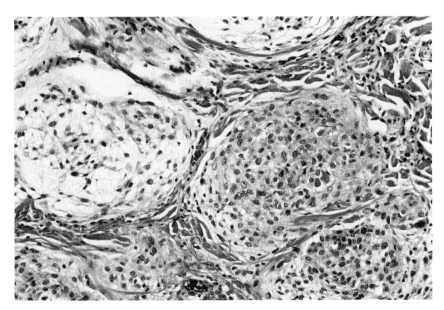

Fig. 122. *Neurothekeoma.* (Reprinted with permission from F. Enzinger and S. W. Weiss, Soft Tissue Tumors, 2nd edn, 1988, Mosby, St. Louis)

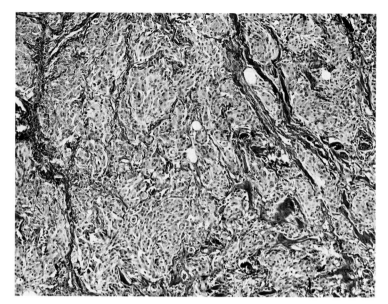

Fig. 123. *Ectopic meningioma*

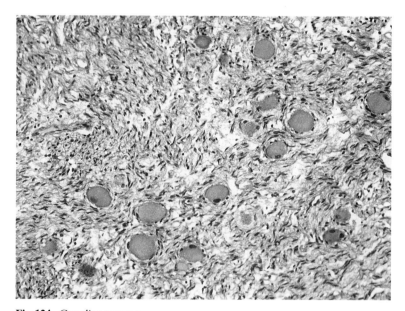

Fig. 124. *Ganglioneuroma*

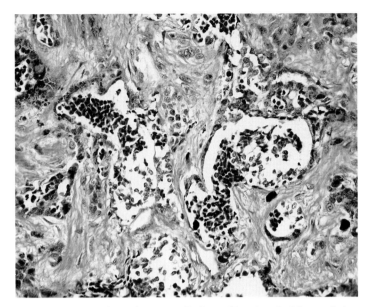

Fig. 125. *Pigmented neuroectodermal tumour of infancy.* (Reprinted with permission from F. Enzinger and S. W. Weiss, Soft Tissue Tumors, 2nd edn, 1988, Mosby, St. Louis)

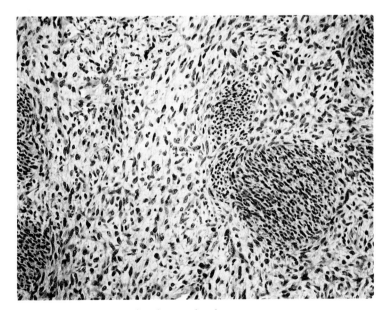

Fig. 126. *Malignant peripheral nerve sheath tumour*

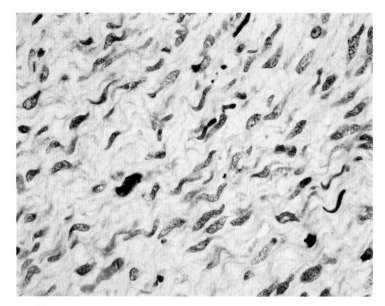

Fig. 127. *Malignant peripheral nerve sheath tumour*

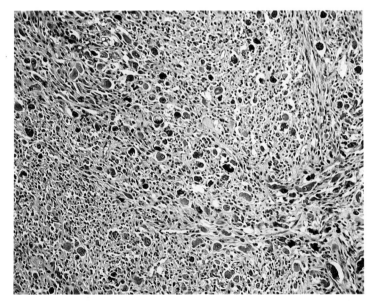

Fig. 128. *Malignant peripheral nerve sheath tumour with rhabdomyoblastic differentiation (malignant Triton tumour)*

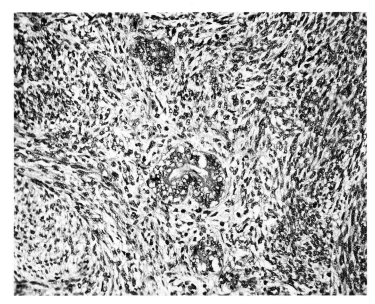

Fig. 129. *Malignant peripheral nerve sheath tumour with glandular differentiation*

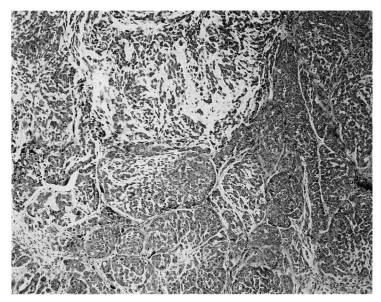

Fig. 130. *Epithelioid malignant peripheral nerve sheath tumour.* (Reprinted with permission from F. Enzinger and S. W. Weiss, Soft Tissue Tumors, 2nd edn, 1988, Mosby, St. Louis)

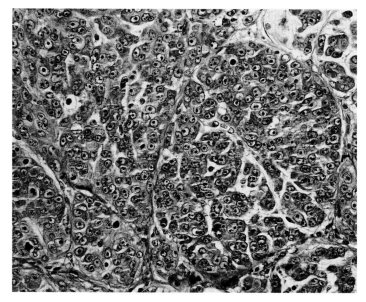

Fig. 131. *Epithelioid malignant peripheral nerve sheath tumour.* (Reprinted with permission from F. Enzinger and S. W. Weiss, Soft Tissue Tumors, 2nd edn, 1988, Mosby, St. Louis)

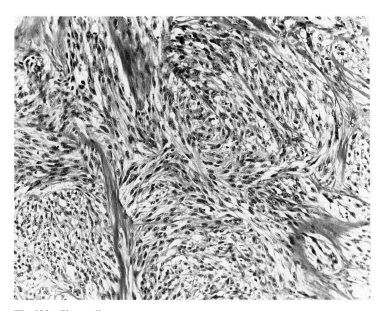

Fig. 132. *Clear cell sarcoma*

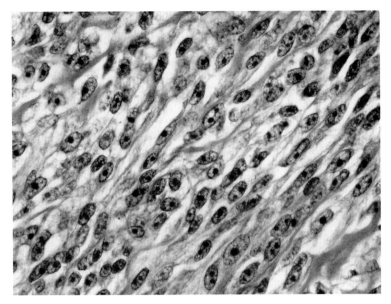

Fig. 133. *Clear cell sarcoma*

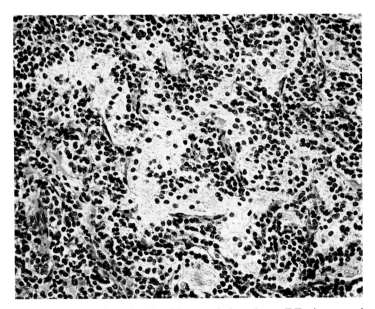

Fig. 134. *Neuroblastoma.* (Reprinted with permission from F. Enzinger and S. W. Weiss, Soft Tissue Tumors, 2nd edn, 1988, Mosby, St. Louis)

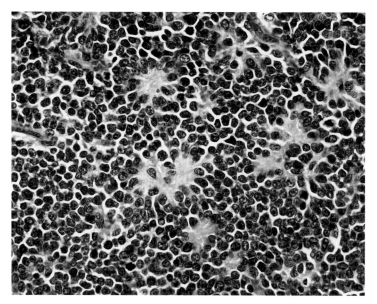

Fig. 135. *Neuroblastoma.* (Reprinted with permission from F. Enzinger and S. W. Weiss, Soft Tissue Tumors, 2nd edn, 1988, Mosby, St. Louis)

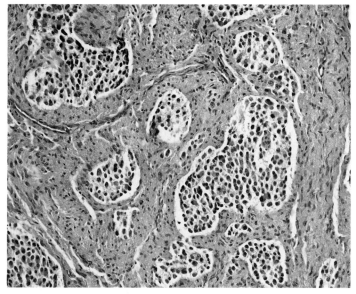

Fig. 136. *Ganglioneuroblastoma.* (Reprinted with permission from F. Enzinger and S. W. Weiss, Soft Tissue Tumors, 2nd edn, 1988, Mosby, St. Louis)

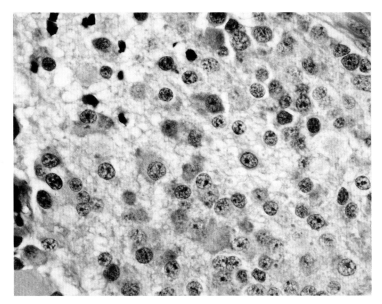

Fig. 137. *Ganglioneuroblastoma*

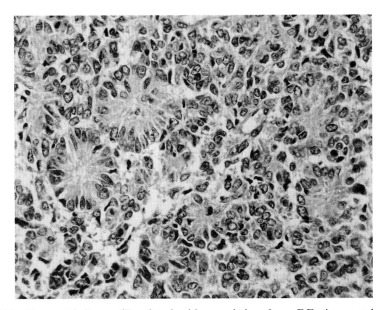

Fig. 138. *Neuroepithelioma.* (Reprinted with permission from F. Enzinger and S. W. Weiss, Soft Tissue Tumors, 2nd edn, 1988, Mosby, St. Louis)

120

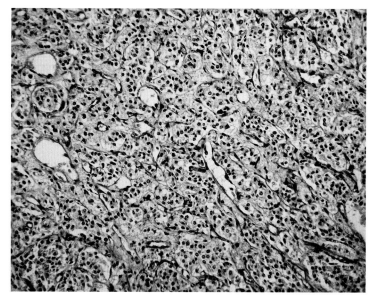

Fig. 139. *Paraganglioma.* Carotid body

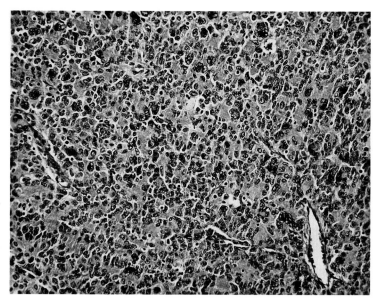

Fig. 140. *Malignant paraganglioma.* (Reprinted with permission from F. Enzinger and S. W. Weiss, Soft Tissue Tumors, 2nd edn, 1988, Mosby, St. Louis)

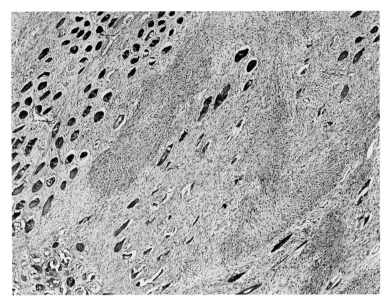

Fig. 141. *Myositis ossificans*

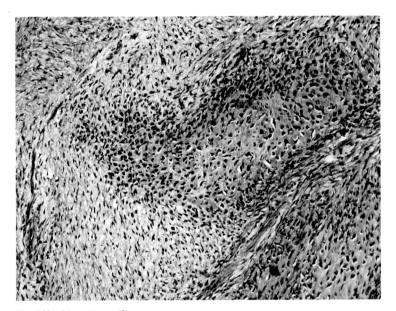

Fig. 142. *Myositis ossificans*

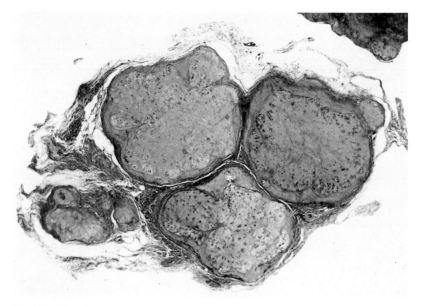

Fig. 143. *Chondroma*

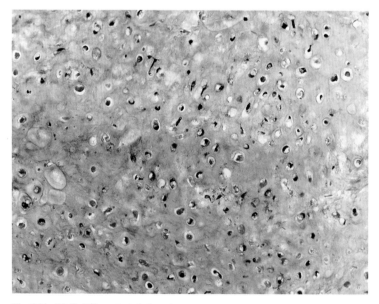

Fig. 144. *Well-differentiated chondrosarcoma*

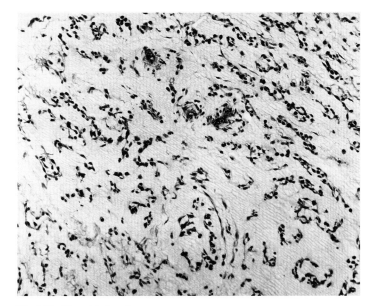

Fig. 145. *Myxoid chondrosarcoma*

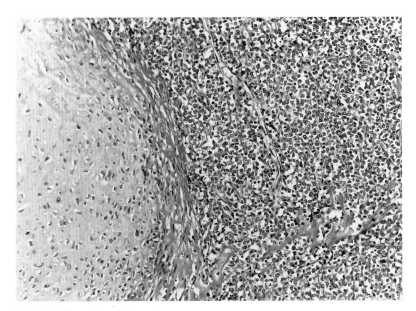

Fig. 146. *Mesenchymal chondrosarcoma*

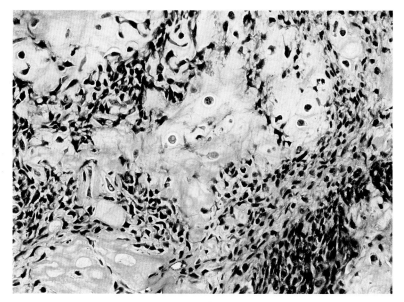

Fig. 147. *Dedifferentiated chondrosarcoma*

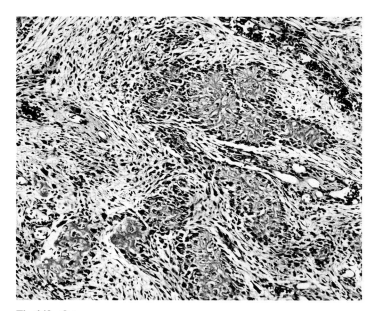

Fig. 148. *Osteosarcoma*

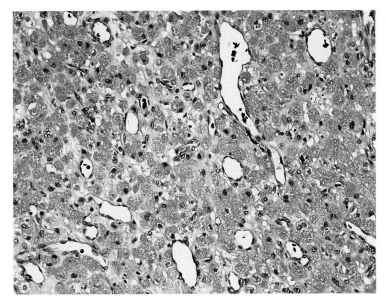

Fig. 149. *Congenital granular cell tumour*

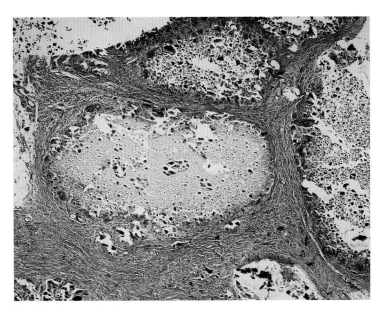

Fig. 150. *Tumoral calcinosis*

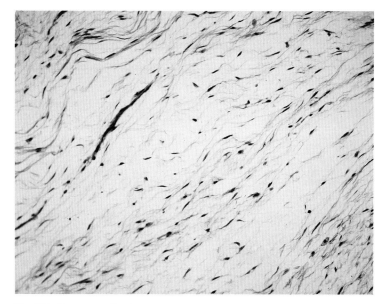

Fig. 151. *Intramuscular myxoma*

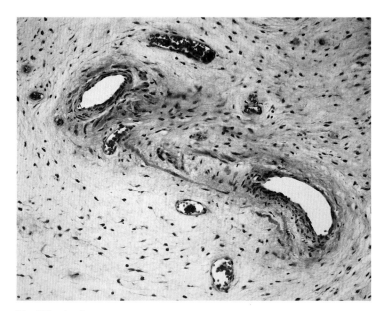

Fig. 152. *Angiomyxoma*

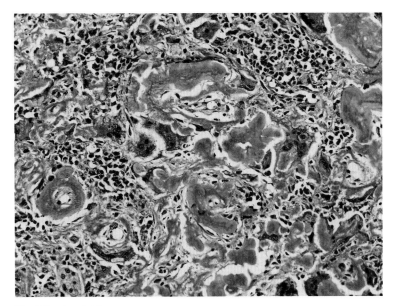

Fig. 153. *Amyloid tumour*

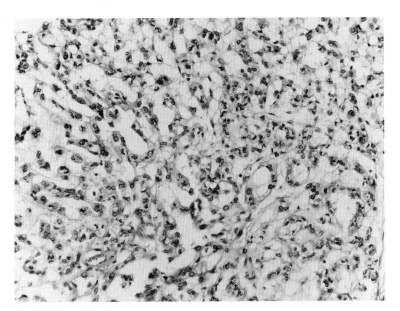

Fig. 154. *Parachordoma*

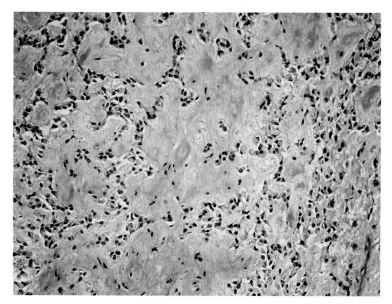

Fig. 155. *Ossifying fibromyxoid tumour.* (Reprinted with permission from Am J Surg Pathol 13: 817, 1989)

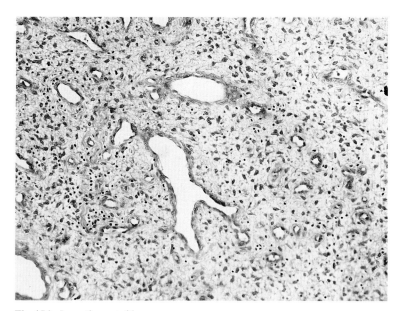

Fig. 156. *Juvenile angiofibroma*

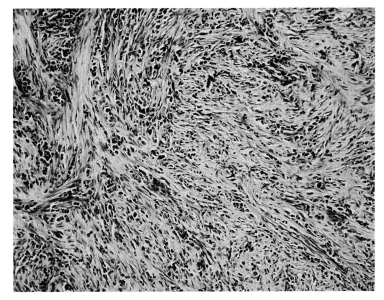

Fig. 157. *Inflammatory myofibroblastic tumour*

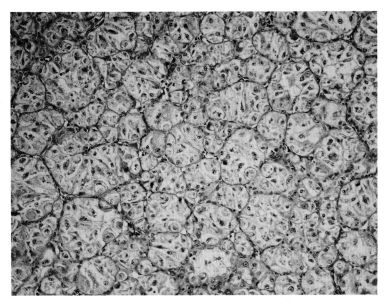

Fig. 158. *Alveolar soft part sarcoma*

130

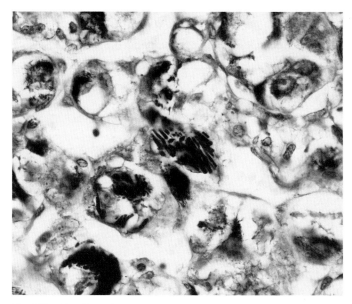

Fig. 159. *Alveolar soft part sarcoma.* Periodic acid-Schiff-positive, diastase-resistant crystals

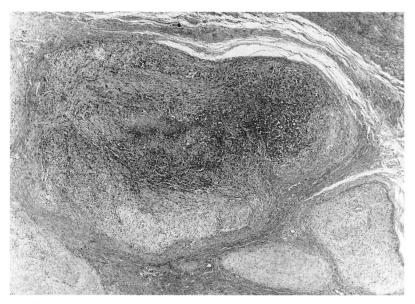

Fig. 160. *Epithelioid sarcoma*

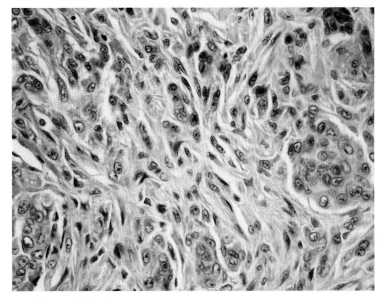

Fig. 161. *Epithelioid sarcoma*

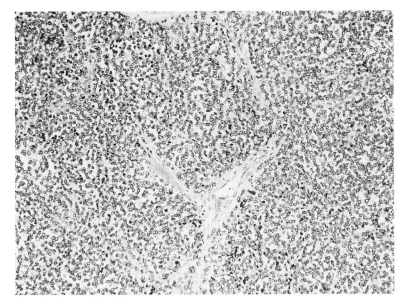

Fig. 162. *Extraskeletal Ewing sarcoma*

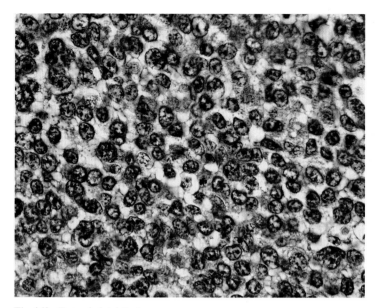

Fig. 163. *Extraskeletal Ewing sarcoma*

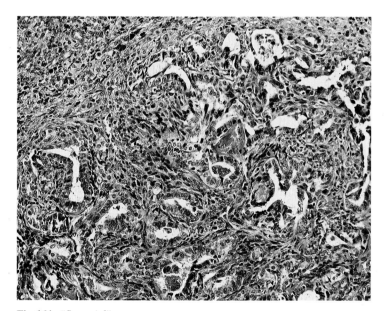

Fig. 164. *"Synovial" sarcoma*

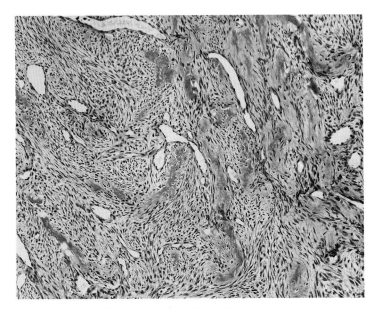

Fig. 165. *"Synovial" sarcoma, monophasic fibrous type*

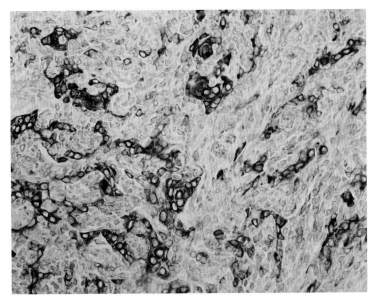

Fig. 166. *"Synovial" sarcoma.* Intense cytokeratin immunoreactivity of glandular component (peroxidase-antiperoxidase). (Reprinted with permission from F. Enzinger and S. W. Weiss, Soft Tissue Tumors, 2nd edn, 1988, Mosby, St. Louis)

134

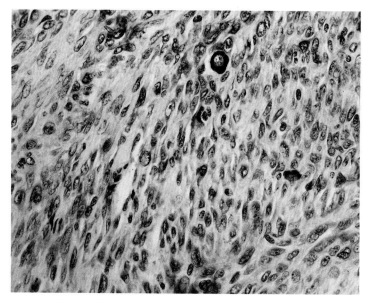

Fig.167. *"Synovial" sarcoma.* Cytokeratin in spindle cell component (peroxidase-antiperoxidase). (Reprinted with permission from F. Enzinger and S. W. Weiss, Soft Tissue Tumors, 2nd edn, 1988, Mosby, St. Louis)

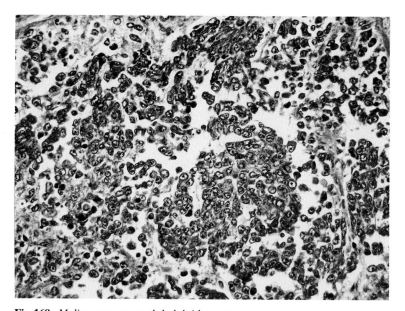

Fig.168. *Malignant extrarenal rhabdoid tumour*

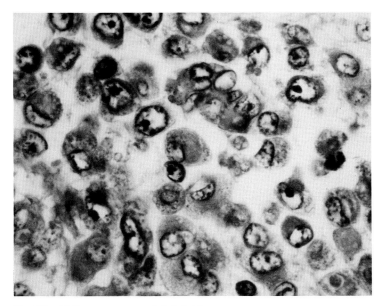

Fig. 169. *Malignant extrarenal rhabdoid tumour*

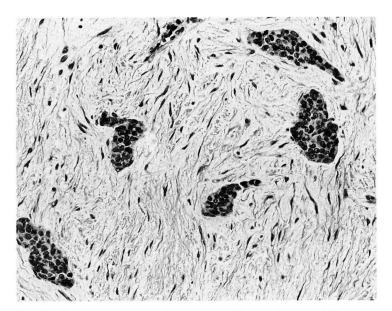

Fig. 170. *Desmoplastic small cell tumour of children and young adults*

Subject Index